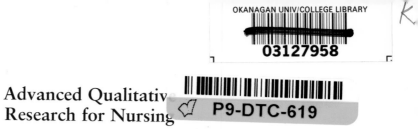

Advanced Qualitativ
Research for Nursing

DATE DUE

NOV 2 1 2003	
JAN 1 5 2004	

BRODART   Cat. No. 23-221

Advanced Qualitative Research for Nursing

Edited by

JOANNA LATIMER
PhD, RGN, BA(Hons)
Cardiff University

Blackwell
Science

© 2003 by Blackwell Science Ltd,
a Blackwell Publishing Company
Editorial Offices:
Osney Mead, Oxford OX2 0EL, UK
  Tel: +44 (0)1865 206206
Blackwell Science, Inc., 350 Main Street,
Malden, MA 02148-5018, USA
  Tel: +1 781 388 8250
Iowa State Press, a Blackwell Publishing
Company, 2121 State Avenue, Ames, Iowa
50014-8300, USA
  Tel: +1 515 292 0140
Blackwell Publishing Asia Pty Ltd,
550 Swanston Street, Carlton South,
Victoria 3053, Australia
  Tel: +61 (0)3 9347 0300
Blackwell Wissenschafts Verlag,
Kurfürstendamm 57, 10707 Berlin,
Germany
  Tel: +49 (0)30 32 79 060

First published 2003 by
Blackwell Science Ltd

Library of Congress
Cataloging-in-Publication Data
is available

ISBN 0-632-05946-X

A catalogue record for this title is available
from the British Library

Set in 11/14 Sabon
by DP Photosetting, Aylesbury, Bucks
Printed and bound in Great Britain by
TJ International Ltd, Padstow, Cornwall

For further information on
Blackwell Publishing, visit our website:
www.blackwellpublishing.com

Contents

Preface

Advanced Qualitative Research offers essays on qualitative methodologies developed to research nursing practice and health care in ways which reflect their complexity. The work represented here is international and interdisciplinary. The approaches discussed produce research which is both theoretically informed and relevant. At the same time, the ideas offered help rewrite what can be counted as relevant not just to nurses and patients, but also to the organisation of health care more generally.

I was once a nurse, and am now a practising social scientist. My work, like that of colleagues writing in this book, has been at pains to make visible the socio-political conditions under which nurses practise and which nurses' practices help to (re)produce. But the authors here have each attempted to go further than that.

Nursing research has been accused by one of the most highly respected of methodological writers of being overly romantic. This means that naiveté over methodology in nursing research can detract from its validity. Some nursing research is certainly seen to be driven by a professionalising agenda. In contrast, critical nursing research, as methodologically and theoretically sound as it may be, is at risk of leaving out some of the story about what nurses accomplish. This challenge requires different kinds of approaches which go beyond the critical.

For most of the authors, nursing and health care are about keeping the other, and their otherness, in mind. In many ways, health care practices engage people in relations where what is at stake *is* otherness. This is to stress the uniqueness of any illness for the person and their loved ones, and acknowledge the invisible and the inexpressible. The methodologies in this volume reflect this:

they are designed to make visible what is so easily marginalised or left implicit.

While to recognise our debt to social phenomena is not to lessen the authenticity of people as persons, selves emerge in our methodologies as socially located subjects. Rather than individual isolates, they remain experiencing and sentient beings. Consequently, as methodologically rigorous and epistemologically complex as the following articles are, they all keep sight of a key issue for any research on nursing and health care: an engagement as, and with, persons.

We would like to thank our editors for the opportunity to publish this collection, and the book's reviewers for their support and insightful comments.

JL

List of contributors

Dr Lioness Ayres is Assistant Professor, University of Wisconsin–Madison School of Nursing, USA. Lioness received her PhD in nursing science from the University of Illinois at Chicago in 1998, where her research into family caregiving received a Dean's Award. From 1998 to 2000, she was a postdoctoral fellow in family nursing at the Oregon Health Sciences University. She is currently conducting research into farm families' response to the injury and subsequent disability of a family member. Publications include: 'Narratives of family caregiving: four story types', *Research in Nursing and Health* (2000) **23**: 359–71; 'Narratives of family caregiving: the process of making meaning', *Research in Nursing and Health* (2000) **23**: 424–34; 'The virtual text and the growth of meaning in qualitative research' (with S. Poirier), *Research in Nursing and Health* (1996) **19**: 163–9.

Dr Kate Gerrish is Reader in Nursing Practice Development, School of Nursing and Midwifery, at the University of Sheffield, UK. Kate practised for a number of years in acute care and community nursing in the UK and Zambia before moving into the field of nurse education. Her main research interests are in the areas of multicultural health with a particular focus on the interplay of policy and practice; the interface between nurse education and practice; and the organisation and delivery of community nursing services. Kate is co-editor of *Ethnicity and Health* and a member of the editorial board of the *Journal of Advanced Nursing*. Publications include: *Nursing for a Multi-ethnic Society* (with C. Husband and J. Mackenzie; Open University Press, 1996); 'The nature and effect of communication difficulties arising from interactions between district nurses and South Asian patients and their carers', *Journal of*

Advanced Nursing (2001) **33**(5): 566–74; 'Whither nursing? Discourses underlying the attribution of master's level performance in nursing (with P. Ashworth and M. McManus), *Journal of Advanced Nursing* (2001) **34**(5): 621–8; 'Individualised care: its conceptualisation and practice within a multi-ethnic society', *Journal of Advanced Nursing* (2000) **32**(1): 91–9; 'Researching ethnic diversity in the British National Health Service: methodological and practical concerns', *Journal of Advanced Nursing* (2000) **31**(4): 918–25; 'Teamwork in primary health care: an evaluation of the contribution of integrated community nursing teams', *Health and Social Care in the Community* (1999) **7**(5): 367–75; 'Inequalities in service provision: an examination of institutional influences on the provision of district nursing care to minority ethnic communities', *Journal of Advanced Nursing* (1999) **30**(6): 1263–71; 'Being a "marginal native": dilemmas of the participant observer', *Nurse Researcher* (1997) **5**(1): 25–34.

Dr Joanna Latimer was a Ward Sister before being awarded a research fellowship by the Scottish Home and Health Department to study at the University of Edinburgh. Since then she has been Senior Research Fellow in Nursing, and Research Officer in Social Gerontology (Keele University), before joining the sociology group in the newly formed School of Social Science at Cardiff University. Joanna is associate editor of *Work, Gender and Organisation*, and a founder member of both the Centre for the Study of Knowledge in Practice (Cardiff University) and the Centre for Social Theory and Technology (Keele University). She has published widely in nursing and in social science, including her ethnography of acute medical care, *The Conduct of Care: Understanding nursing practice* (Blackwell Science, 2000). She is currently working on two new books: an ethnography of multidisciplinary work in elderly care and a book on the sociology of nursing and medicine. Her other publications include *Interdisciplinary Perspectives on Health Policy and Practice: Competing Interests or Complementary Interpretations?* (with J. Robinson, M. Avis and M. Traynor; Harcourt Brace, 1999); 'Socialising disease: medical categories and inclusion of the aged', *Sociological Review* (2000) **48**(3): 383–407; 'The dark at the bottom of the stair: participation and performance of older people in hospital', *Medical Anthropology Quarterly* (1999) **13**(2): 186–

213; 'Organising context: nurses' assessments of older people in an acute medical unit', *Nursing Inquiry* (1998) **5**(1): 43–57; 'Giving patients a future: the constituting of classes in an acute medical unit', *Sociology of Health and Illness* (1997) **19**(2): 160–78; 'The nursing process re-examined: diffusion or translation?', *Journal of Advanced Nursing* (1995) **22**: 213–20.

Dr Carl May is Professor of Medical Sociology in the Centre for Health Services Research at the University of Newcastle-upon-Tyne, UK. Carl has a long-standing interest in the application of qualitative research techniques to evaluation studies, focusing increasingly on the employment of formative process evaluation methods within clinical trials. His doctoral research on nurse–patient relationships in terminal care was followed by appointments at the Universities of Edinburgh, Liverpool and Manchester between 1990 and 2001, and led to a series of studies on the changing contexts of professional–patient interaction and the social construction of chronic disease and incapacity in primary care. In parallel, since 1996 he has investigated the social production of knowledge and practice around new information and communications technologies in health care. He has researched and published widely on these topics, with studies funded by the Medical Research Council, Economic and Social Research Council, Department of Health and other agencies. He has published in *Acta Sociologica, Family Practice, Journal of Advanced Nursing, Journal of Telemedicine and Telecare, Social Science and Medicine, Sociology, Sociology of Health and Illness* amongst others. Carl May was the recipient of the Diana E. Forsythe Award for Social Science Research of the American Medical Informatics Association in 2001.

Dr Siobhan Nelson is Associate Professor, School of Postgraduate Nursing, University of Melbourne, Australia. Siobhan, a registered nurse and historian, is editor of the influential international journal *Nursing Inquiry* (Blackwell). Publications include: *Say Little Do Much: Nursing, Nuns and Hospitals in the Nineteenth Century* (Pennsylvania University Press, 2001); *A Genealogy of Care of the Sick* (Nursing Praxis Press, 2000); 'Insiders and outsiders in writing history' in *A Question of Ethics: Personal Perspectives* (History

Institute, Vic., Inc., 1999, pp. 38–45); 'From salvation to civics: service to the sick in nursing discourse', *Social Science and Medicine* (2001) **53**: 1217–25; 'A fork in the road: nursing history versus history of nursing', *Nursing History Review* (2002) **9**; 'Hair-dressing and nursing: presentation of self in Colonial Sydney', *The Collegian* (2001) 8(2): 28–31; 'Déjà vu and the regulation of nursing', *Australian Journal of Advanced Nursing* (1999) **16**(4): 29–35; 'Entering the professional domain: the making of the modern nurse in 17th century France', *Nursing History Review* (1999) 7: 171–88; 'How do we write a nursing history of disease?', *Health and History* (1998) 1(1): 43–7; 'Reading nursing history', *Nursing Inquiry* (1997) 4(4): 229–36; 'Pastoral care and moral government: early nineteenth century nursing and solutions to the Irish question', *Journal of Advanced Nursing* (1997) 26(1): 6–14; 'Holistic nursing: the re-emergence of the light', *Nursing Inquiry* (1995) 2: 36–43.

Dr Judith M. Parker is Professor, School of Post-Graduate Nursing, University of Melbourne, Australia, and Managing Editor of *Nursing Inquiry*. Judith has published extensively in the fields of her major research interests which are cancer nursing and palliative care and the psychodynamics of customary nursing practices. She is particularly interested in the changes currently under way within the health care system and the implications of new models of practice for the education of health professionals generally.

Dr Suzanne Poirier is Professor of Literature and Medical Education at the University of Illinois at Chicago, USA, where she teaches courses in literature to medical students. Suzanne is co-author with Lioness Ayres of *Stories of Family Caregiving: Reconsiderations of Theory, Literature, and Life* (Nursing Centre Press, forthcoming). Her current research is a book-length study of physicians' memoirs published since 1965.

Dr Mary Ellen Purkis is Associate Professor of Nursing, University of Victoria, Canada. Mary Ellen has undertaken numerous field studies of nursing in a range of practice settings including surgery, public health and home care. Her latest study explores the concepts of capacity and continuity for people with cancer. Publications include: 'Governing the health of populations: the child, the clinic and the "conversation"', in V. Hayes & L. Young (eds) *Health Promotion and Nursing Practice* (Los Angeles: F.A. Davis, 2001, pp. 190–206); 'Managing home nursing care: visibility, accountability and exclusion', *Nursing Inquiry* (2001) 8(3): 141–50; 'Embracing technology: an exploration of the effects of writing nursing', *Nursing Inquiry* (1999) 6(3): 147–56; 'The "social determinants" of practice? A critical analysis of health promoting discourse', *Canadian Journal of Nursing Research* (1997) **29**(1): 47–62; 'Nursing in quality space: technologies governing experiences of care', *Nursing Inquiry* (1996) **3**: 101–11.

Dr Trudy Rudge is Associate Professor in the School of Nursing, Flinders University, Adelaide, Australia. Trudy is the editor of Post-Graduate Update in *Nursing Inquiry*. Publications include: 'Discourse, metaphor and body boundaries', in J. Lawler (ed.) *The Body in Nursing: A Collection of Views* (Churchill Livingstone, 1997, pp. 75–93); 'Procedure manuals and textually mediated death', *Nursing Inquiry* (2001) **8**: 264–72 (with B. Quested); 'Reawakenings? A discourse analysis of the recovery from schizophrenia after medication change', *Australian and New Zealand Journal of Mental Health Nursing* (2001) **10**: 66–76 (with K. Morse); 'Situating wound management: technoscience, dressings and "other" skins', *Nursing Inquiry* (1999) **6**: 167–77; 'Skin as cover: the discursive framing of metaphors in burns care', *Nursing Inquiry* (1998) **5**: 228–37; 'Unpacking my(our) clinical practice ... again' (editorial), *Contemporary Nurse* (1996) **5**: 144–8; 'Nursing wounds: exploring the presence of abjection in nursing practice', *Nursing Inquiry* (1996) **3**(4): 250–1.

Dr Margarete Sandelowski is Professor of Nursing and Director of the Annual Summer Institutes in Qualitative Research at the University of North Carolina at Chapel Hill School of Nursing (USA). She has published extensively in both nursing and social science journals and books in the areas of reproductive technology, technology in nursing, and qualitative methodology. She is a Fellow in the American Academy of Nursing, Assistant Editor of *Research in Nursing and Health*, and North American Editor of *Nursing Inquiry*. Her book *With Child in Mind: Studies of the Personal*

Encounter with Infertility (University of Pennsylvania Press, 1993) was awarded a national book prize from the American Anthropological Association. Her latest book is *Devices and Desires: Gender, Technology, and American Nursing* (University of North Carolina Press, 2000). She is currently principal investigator of a study, funded for five years by the National Institute for Nursing Research, National Institutes of Health, to develop analytical techniques for conducting qualitative metasyntheses.

Dr Jan Savage is Senior Research Fellow at the Royal College of Nursing Institute, London, UK, where she leads on the 'New roles and technologies' theme of the Institute's research strategy. As both a nurse and an anthropologist, Jan is interested in applying anthropological theory to the study of nursing, particularly in terms of developing methodological approaches for articulating the less tangible aspects of nursing practice. Publications include: *Nursing Intimacy: An Ethnographic Approach to Nurse–Patient Interaction* (Scutari, 1995); 'Ethnography and health care', *British Medical Journal* (2000) **321**: 1400–2; 'The "culture" of culture in National Health Service policy implementation', *Nursing Inquiry* (2000) **7**: 230–38; 'One voice, different tunes: issues raised by dual analysis of a segment of qualitative data', *Journal of Advanced Nursing* (2000) **31**(6): 1493–1500; 'Participative observation: standing in the shoes of others?', *Qualitative Health Research* (2000) **10**(3): 324–39; 'Gestures of resistance: the nurse's body in contested space', *Nursing Inquiry* (1997) **4**: 237–45.

Dr Michael Traynor is Senior Lecturer, Centre for Policy in Nursing Research, London School of Hygiene and Tropical Medicine, UK. Michael's publications include: *Exemplary Research in Nursing and Midwifery* (edited with A-M. Rafferty; Routledge, 2002); *Managerialism and Nursing: Beyond Profession and Oppression* (Routledge, 1999); *Interdisciplinary Perspectives on Health Policy and Practice: Competing Interests or Complementary Interpretations?* (with J. Robinson, M. Avis and J. Latimer; Churchill Livingstone/Harcourt Brace, 1999); 'Endogenous and exogenous research? Findings from a bibliometric study of UK nursing research' (with A-M. Rafferty and G. Lewison), *Journal of Advanced Nursing* (2001) **34**(2): 212–22; 'Purity, conversion and the evidence-based movements', *Health* (2000) **4**(2): 139–58; 'Postmodern research: no grounding or privilege, just free-floating trouble making', *Nursing Inquiry* (1997) **4**: 99–107; *Nursing Research and the Higher Education Context: A Second Working Paper* (with A-M. Rafferty; Centre for Policy in Nursing Research, London School of Hygiene and Tropical Medicine, March 1998); 'Context, convergence and contingency' (editorial; with A-M. Rafferty) *Journal of Health Services Research and Policy* (1998) **3**(4): 195; 'Building and benchmarking research capacity for nursing' (guest editorial; with A-M. Rafferty), *Nursing Times Research* (1999) **4**(1): 5–7; 'Nurse education in an international context: the contribution of contingency' (with A-M. Rafferty), *International Journal of Nursing Studies* (1999) **36**(1): 85–91; ' "Do nurses need degrees?" Questions & Answers Section' (with A-M. Rafferty), *Journal of Health Services Research and Policy* (1999) **4**(3); 'Nursing and the RAE: past, present and future' (with A-M. Rafferty), *Journal of Advanced Nursing* (1999) **30**(1): 186–92; 'The problem of dissemination: evidence and ideology', *Nursing Inquiry* (1999) **6**: 187–97.

Dr John Wiltshire is Reader in English at La Trobe University, Melbourne, Australia. Since the publication of *Samuel Johnson in the Medical World* (1991) and *Jane Austen and the Body: 'The Picture of Health'*, John has worked with Judith Parker on a number of projects mainly concerned with aspects of narrative formation by nurses and patients. Their publications include 'The handover: three modes of nursing knowledge', in G. Gray and R. Pratt (eds) *Scholarship in the Discipline of Nursing* (Churchill Livingstone, 1995) and 'Containing abjection in nursing: the end of shift handover as site of containment', *Nursing Inquiry* (1996) **3**(1).

CHAPTER 1

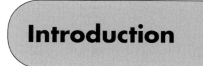

Introduction

Joanna Latimer

This book brings together contributions from Australia, Canada, the UK and the USA. It consists of a collection of empirically based articles presenting and explaining approaches to qualitative research by authors at the front-line in academic nursing and health services research. In addition, the book is interdisciplinary – each chapter brings together ideas coming from a range of disciplines, such as anthropology, sociology, history, literary and psycho-analytic theory, nursing and cultural studies.

The aim of the book is to show how qualitative methodologies can produce rigorous and relevant understandings about nursing practice and patienthood. This is important because qualitative methodologies are often viewed within the competitive world of health research as *epistemologically* inferior to 'more positive' approaches. So that while there are many excellent 'how to do it' books on qualitative research methods for nurses, their epistemo-logical grounds are usually treated to a separate account from the presentation of methods. Further, methods books in nursing often present methodologies as derivative or predeveloped.

Many of the chapters in the current book take a different position over methodology. First, the authors present research developments that make their theoretical grounds explicit and integral. Second, they presume that the very notion of *applying* a method may be inconsistent with researching how a practical discipline, like nur-sing, occurs. Thus, in contrast to research textbooks for nurses, the current book features nursing as *dynamic practice* and offers methodological approaches that are themselves dynamic and creative.

Rather than simply showing how to apply an approach, each chapter moves between ways of researching and ideas for understanding. To do this, each author draws on and develops ideas deriving from different disciplines. For example, Sandelowski (Chapter 10) and Nelson (Chapter 11) each make different aspects of the materiality of nurses' worlds (dressings, nursing records, technologies and other artefacts) explicit and central, rather than implicit and peripheral. They focus on how materials in nursing can be researched and how their significance, for understanding the socio-cultural context of nursing, or for illuminating nurses' accomplishments, can be 'read'. But each author's approach to how we can read materials draws on very different theoretical understandings. On the one hand, Sandelowski draws together ideas deriving from the material culture tradition with those coming from anthropology and sociology, while Nelson explicates a critical historical approach.

In addition, as well as offering an interdisciplinary approach to researching nursing, each chapter also helps redraw the boundaries around what constitutes an appropriate clinical topic. The major funders of health research usually want studies that *they* can account for. The kind of research that is easily accounted for promises practical results with, clear clinical relevance. But, what counts as clinical is predefined in ways which favour the heroic, the functional, the clear and distinct. The implicit and marginalised aspects of clinical practice are transformed in this book, into proper topics for nursing research, as well as important resources in its methodology. For example, Savage (Chapter 4) rethinks the embodied nature of social being, of nursing and of patienthood, to re-place the body in research on nursing. While Purkis (Chapter 3) and Rudge (Chapter 9), refuting any simplistic notion that nursing is merely the *application* of knowledge or the *delivery* of care packages, offer approaches that focus the dynamic and interactive aspects of nurses' encounters with patients. And Parker and Wiltshire (Chapter 6) foreground a taken-for-granted practice: the nursing handover. By drawing together psychoanalytic theory with a literary approach to textual analysis they are able to reveal the importance of the handover to nursing practice.

In these ways, each approach offered in the book helps make visible the rationality and meaning of aspects of practice which might remain hidden to functionalist evaluations of nursing procedures and processes. But the authors face up to a further dilemma that confronts anyone researching nursing practice.

There is an unwritten insistence that research on nursing must display an allegiance to the humanist tradition that informs most nursing theory. Consequently, the mainstream qualitative tradition in nursing research gets caught by the demand for positive knowledge together with overly romantic notions about the experiencing individual (Silverman, 1989). The result can be research that is sociologically naive.

The authors of the chapters that follow confront this dilemma. At the same time as they treat the world of health care as a political and contested site, they centralise a concern with nursing and health care as engaging people as persons. A key feature of the book is therefore to offer ways to research nursing as located in socio-cultural relations at the same time as nurses, and researchers, are featured as persons embedded *in relations* with others. Indeed, otherness emerges as of central concern to nursing practice. This is not to suggest that regard for the other is straightforward, as May, Savage, Gerrish and Traynor illustrate in their chapters. Nurses', and researchers', engagements with the other cannot be taken for granted; on the contrary, nurses' and researchers' relations are mediated by many social and cultural influences in ways which nursing theory does not always admit to. Thus, many of the chapters, in their different ways, help make the problem of otherness a central concern for clinical practice and for the development of appropriate methodologies for researching nursing and health care.

Structure of the book

Recognising that nursing and researching are both dynamic practices changes everything. First, it means that time, space and context have to be taken seriously. Second, it means that we have to face up to the fact that nursing and researching are interactive. Third, it means that we will be flying in the face of a dominant research paradigm in health research which stresses the need for knowledge which helps us predict, control and standardise.

The book is divided into five parts: fields, selves, stories, texts and materials. Each of these headings signals a methodological approach that integrates with features particular to nursing practice. The chapters under each heading present methodological developments to reflect the dynamics and politics of nursing practice and nursing research. In presenting methodologies consistent with nursing practice and epistemology, the book not only enables a better representation of nursing work, but also makes an important contribution to social science.

Fields

In their chapters, May (Chapter 2) and Purkis (Chapter 3) both draw out how the field, defined by the researcher's approach to it, is both a lived as well as a contested and political site. It does not 'exist', but rather is constructed by the very ways in which it is 'thought' by a research project. And this way of thinking connects to the very ways in which nursing and health care are being imagined – to the assumptions and taken-for-granted ideas which underpin a research study.

To put it another way, a research project 'thinks' the field up in ways that have distinct political effects. On the one hand, as May shows, one political effect of the way in which a research project 'thinks' the field, is how it constructs particular kinds of power relations between the researcher and the researched. Gerrish also addresses this sensitive issue in her chapter on participant observation, and connects it to how the researcher can conduct him or herself reflexively. On the other hand, as Purkis illuminates, the ways in which the field is imagined reflects the assumptions underpinning the ways in which *nursing* is being imagined.

In Chapter 2, then, May explores the critical issue of the place of qualitative methodology in evaluation research. He helps us to understand how a field is made up of subjects, including the researcher, whose relations to each other are constructed through the research approach. In this way, drawing on the work of Michel Foucault, May elucidates the research approach itself as a complex political and epistemological act. His starting point is how evaluation research usually deletes questions about the politics of research and the location of the researcher's subjectivity. In particular it removes any notion that the researcher is in any more than a functional relation to the researched. May argues that the rhetorics of evaluation research thus present the research approach as 'a self-evident technical process in which methods are "objective" and asocial'. In contrast, his own chapter explicates *how* the subjects of evaluation methodology are constituted by the research process in a political relation to each other. Specifically, the qualitative researcher elicits respondents' accounts in ways which contribute to the survey and grading (or evaluation) of their practices.

May's dilemma is that a qualitative approach to knowledge generation is increasingly being drawn into the evaluation of health service provision in ways that are problematic because of the ways evaluation research (ER) erases these issues of politics and reflexivity. He shows how, once the lid is off and principles of reflexivity are applied to the political context of ER, we can begin to understand how 'qualitative inquiry, constituted as an element of ER, mobilises power and transforms experience through the exercise of surveillance'. May thus extends the debate initiated by Silverman and Gubrium (1989) over how the qualitative researcher can respond to being constituted as an 'accomplice in other people's political projects' (p. 2).

In the context of multiple possibilities for conduct, and in the absence of coercion, it becomes crucial that social actors attend to the issue of persuasion (Fernandez, 1986). If it is accepted that there are, in any social context, multiple possibilities for interpretation, social life, in order to become organised, can be considered in terms of the advancement of different sets of interests, including persuading other people to 'see' something in one way rather than another. However, what makes up the capacity to be persuasive is connected to 'grounds' (Lyotard, 1984): persuasiveness is inter-related with authority, not just the authority invested by status and position, but the authority which comes from drawing on particular kinds of grounds.

Focusing on health promotion as central to discourse in contemporary health care, Purkis demonstrates how nurses' activities do not simply entail unproblematic application of knowledge or the delivery of services to patients. Purkis draws on anthropologist James Fernandez to illustrate when encounters between a nurse and her patient need to be understood as 'argumentation'. In this way her approach constitutes patient and nurse as knowledgeable subjects, whose encounters help accomplish health promotion through forms of persuasion.

Specifically, Purkis attends to how the field is made up of multiple possible meanings and interests, and that research on nursing needs methods for exploring patients' and nurses' competing understandings and representations of events. The chapter begins with an extended critique of research which does not take the dynamic nature of practice seriously. Purkis suggests that 'the lack of theoretical attention to power and resistance within a practice discipline such as nursing becomes increasingly frustrating and problematic as one considers the issues of power inherent within [such] examples of health promoting interventions'.

Purkis goes on to offer an approach to both how data is collected, and to its analysis which focuses the accomplished nature of practice as the effect of complex power relations. So that rather than simply focusing on accounts of health-promoting occasions or on abstract representations of their outcomes, Purkis examines these occasions for how they are achieved and for what they achieve. In her example she analyses the text of an encounter between a clinic nurse, a mother and her children. The analysis explores how the clinic nurse uses the results of a 'soft technology' aimed at the 'objective' assessment of an infant's development. The nurse uses the results of her measurements and their interpretation to influence the ways in which the mother parents her infant. But the mother herself has different ideas about her baby's growth, which she grounds in powerful evidence. What Purkis illuminates is how research can capture nurses' attempts to move their patients, and patients' attempts to move nurses back, drawing on different kinds of evidence and grounds. What is at stake is each participant's authority to legitimate action or a proposed action. The chapter ends by suggesting that research which does not take the dynamic and *accomplished* nature of the field seriously, tells us little about the processes through which aims, such as the promotion of health, are, or are not, achieved.

Selves

In Chapter 4, Savage draws on anthropological understandings of embodiment to explicate the process of studying nursing practice through what she has named 'participative observation'. While she argues that nurses' bodies are dextrous, skilled and knowledgeable (Benner, 1984), she explores how nurses' bodies are also implicated in the constitution and circulation of socio-cultural knowledge. Thus at the same time as nurses are involved in 'doing' things, such as sitting on the bed talking to patients, or doing a dressing, or standing at the end of the bed, their bodies can be read as helping to institute particular kinds of relations with others. Put simply, nurses' bodies embody, circulate and communicate meaning.

Drawing on social theorists such as Pierre Bourdieu and Michael Taussig, Savage begins by discussing the role of the body in the generation of knowledge and society. She then illustrates an approach to participation in the field through which the researcher makes explicit the bodily processes that help *produce* nursing practice. Savage makes her own presence and bodily participation and use of all the senses (not just sight) central to the collection and interpretation of data. She shows how it is through making herself aware of her participation in, *or* her inability to participate in these embodied practices, that she can begin to understand what they mean, and what they are in a sense doing, literally and politically, in the production of nursing. So that one aspect of what is being observed is, in a sense, the researcher's own participation as an embodied being. This is important, because as Savage explicates, bodily activity manifests the systems of distinction that help to produce practice. In her approach to research, Savage thus re-places the body as central to nursing, and to understanding how and what nursing practice accomplishes.

Kate Gerrish takes up the theme of reflexivity in her sensitive and informed exploration of the relationship of the researcher to the researched in participant observation (Chapter 5). She focuses on the ethical and substantive dilemmas specific to participant obser-vation of researchers who are also practising nurses. She argues that these dilemmas can be resolved only through making explicit the epistemological grounds of the research approach and through recognising the 'complex and changing nature of field relationships together with the shifting composition of people who interact with the main participants'.

Opting for what she calls a subtle realist approach to guide her, Gerrish explores the tensions between the objectivity of observation as a researcher and the subjectivity of participation as a nurse in the production of nursing understandings and knowledge about patients and their needs. Gerrish considers these issues through exploring her own role as a researcher and a nurse in an ethnographic study of the provision of district nursing care to people from different ethnic backgrounds. She focuses on the place of reflexivity in the research process, the relationship between herself as both researcher and nurse with the research participants, the interface between participant observation and interviewing, and the situational ethics encountered during fieldwork. At the same time, then, as she helps illuminate how a subtle realist approach can help produce rigorous, if partial, knowledge, Gerrish explores the place of the reflexive self in managing the dynamics of the field. She states that 'adopting a subtle realist perspective also made me aware of the need to take into account the personal, social and cultural identities of both the researcher and the researched. One of the methodological challenges of researching ethnicity is that participants will respond in ways they consider appropriate in the context of how they perceive the ethnic identity of the researcher in relation to their own identity'. What emerges in Gerrish's account is the way in which the researcher's capacity to participate in the field is itself, like nursing practice, interactively produced in ways which are mediated by wider socio-cultural issues.

Stories

Parker and Wiltshire's chapter (Chapter 6) reminds us, with Isabel Menzies Lyth, that all those concerned with the organisation of nursing need to attend to the very serious existential and psycho-dynamic dimensions of patienthood and of nursing practice. They argue that story and narrative need to be understood in relation to the maintenance of what Giddens (1991) calls 'ontological security'. On the one hand, the authors construct an argument for an approach to analysing nurses' practices, such as the nursing handover, which helps make visible their often implicit logic and rationality. Through their approach, the handover re-emerges not just as an occasion for the passing on of information, but as a social space in which nurses do the work of 'containing' the existentially pressing aspects of their work. On the other hand, they illuminate why stories are central to the healing of the '*invisible* wounds' (Rudge, 1997) caused by illness and its treatment, such as the surgical construction of a stoma.

Specifically, the authors outline a method of working with story and narrative which enables understanding of some of the complexity surrounding nursing practice and patienthood. They begin by reviewing the ways in which narrative and story are used in nursing research and argue that research that merely reproduces stories is seriously under-theorised so that it fails to fully explain the place of stories in nursing work and in patients' careers. To reconsider the place that story and narrative has in nursing practice and in patienthood, Parker and Wiltshire present an analytic approach which utilises psychoanalytic object-relations theory. They concentrate on one key aspect of object-relations theory, the notion, first advanced by W.R. Bion of 'containing'. They show how to bring this concept to bear in the understanding of two sets of practices within nursing – the traditional end-of-shift handover meeting, and the nursing management of patients with stoma. In their work, story-telling is distinguished as an important, rather than marginal, feature of nurses' and patients' methods for handling those aspects of illness and its treatment that disrupt much more than the biophysical body. Critically, such research findings as those on the handover, help to substantiate the efficacy of aspects of nursing practice, and of the experience of patienthood, whose rationality is normally invisible and which nurses find difficult to justify in the face of pressing efficiency drives.

Weber suggested that the proper project of social science is understanding. However, interpretation of people's actions or accounts is easily rooted in methodological individualism. In contrast, Ayres and Poirier (Chapter 7) describe one approach to the exploration of the meaning of illness through the analysis of stories which avoids such a pitfall. The authors argue that since nurses are often engaged in understanding and treating human responses to health and illness, and since those responses are often highly variable across externally similar circumstances, an understanding of narrative is useful both for nurses and for clinicians. In addition, because nurses, like caregivers, are persons who make meaning out of their experiences in caring for others, they suggest narrative provides a useful approach for understanding and communicating nursing knowledge.

Drawing on a study of family caregiving, the authors present a particular literary approach to the analysis of narratives which attends to voice, content and structure. This approach to the analysis of narratives not only illuminates aspects of caregivers' experience but, crucially, helps to explain why caregivers in externally similar circumstances describe very different meanings for, and affective responses to, caregiving. Specifically, the approach to narrative helps to locate responses to caregiving not merely as the effects of an instrumental rationality, personality or unmediated choice. Rather, responses to caregiving are explained by attending to the caregiver as a social being who is constituted by, and who helps accomplish, a very particular socio-cultural context.

Texts

Michael Traynor begins Chapter 8 by giving an overview of how discourse analysis has been theorised and used as a tool in nursing and health research. His aim is to point to the 'dangers inherent in a discourse analytic approach if it is taken as a way either of accounting for intention or of presenting a stable or undeceived picture of the world, one that is able to perceive the reality beyond ideology'. Drawing together theorists such as Derrida and Rorty, Traynor explicates an approach to discourse analysis that does not deceive itself as being able to detect 'the reality beyond ideology'.

He goes on to exemplify how nurses' and managers' interviews can be analysed and compared as competing discourses, which attempt to settle the complexity and heterogeneity of practice, to produce stable, and distinctive identities. Traynor suggests that this work – of producing the appearance of stable and distinctive identities – rests upon practices of exclusion and othering. But these as power effects are not intended in the usual sense. Rather, Traynor illuminates how it is that nurses and managers are enacting demands coming from the powerful discourses which underpin wider forms of social order and which incite a 'desire' for stability and distinction.

Rudge (Chapter 9) also introduces the notion of desire in her discursive approach to the analysis of ethnographic research material in a burns unit. Her aim in introducing the notion of desire is to suggest that interaction between patient and nurse cannot be approached as if it is the effect of an instrumental, cognitively based rationalism. Her approach is underpinned by an idea that much, much more is at stake as patients and nurses encounter each other.

The chapter draws on research material pertaining to nurse–patient interactions during wound care procedures. These interactions took place during a dressing process that could be protracted if the patient had a large area of skin to (re)cover. Thus, the observations were focused on a practice which is particular to nursing: one that includes the provision of intimate care to patients' bodies together with talk about wounds and their care. In addition, it is a practice that involves terrible pain, fear and other emotion. The chapter reflects on how using ethnographic research material allows wound care to be considered as much more than just a functional event. Rudge offers an approach which illuminates how representations of wound care processes make invisible the constructed nature of the wound care event, as an effect of nurses' and patients' interactions. But through close attention to the texts of these interactions, Rudge shows how nurses and patients can be understood as having competing desires which are or are not brought into alignment. She shows how the tension in the wound care process is an effect of the intersections of the many discourses that go to make it up and how these discourses intersect to constitute 'wound care' in ways that privilege only some possible aspects of wound care practice. Specifically, Rudge illuminates how the way in which wound care is conducted is an effect of discourses which privilege the healing and (re)covering of burnt skin over attention to the recovery of the traumatised person lying beneath the skin.

Materials

Sandelowski, in her comprehensive chapter (Chapter 10), considers the importance of studying the material culture of nursing. She argues that qualitative research in nursing has been conducted almost exclusively with verbal texts so that the material world of the nurse is a hitherto neglected object of nursing inquiry. As well as offering ways to study the material culture of nursing, she illuminates why centralising materials is of particular relevance to nursing as less about cognitive, and more about embodied and material, practices.

The chapter draws on a wide range of literature and research, from nursing, anthropology and sociology as well as material culture studies. It begins with discussion of why the study of materials is important. Sandelowski emphasises how a focus on materials helps to shift old dualisms, such as mind/body or sacred/mundane, in ways that are of particular relevance to nursing. Sandelowski goes on to emphasise that 'the primary concern and problem for any student of material culture [is how to] make matter mean'. She locates methods for making materials mean in different methodologies. For example, she suggests that an ethnomethodological approach to making materials mean, will be different from a structuralist approach. Illustrating each point with rich research scenarios, Sandelowski goes on to identify how to target the physical objects comprising the material world of nursing and suggests ways in which these materials can be read to explore key questions about the meaning and location of nursing in the social world. Specifically, arguing for the 'the exquisite study of the concrete', Sandelowski illuminates how phenomenological reflection on the material and the corporeal can contribute to understandings of patienthood and nursing practice. For example, she explores how the telephone, used in tele-nursing, rematerialises nurse–patient relations and can illuminate how contemporary health care policy and practice are refabricating those relations. Sandelowski goes on to explicate how ethnographic and fieldwork approaches contextualise the use and construction of materials in ways which enhance interpretation of their meaning and their effects. Finally, Sandelowski shows how exploration of media representations of nursing, or the ways in which the materials which make up the life world of nurses have come to stand for the things that they represent, can be used to illuminate the status and character of nursing *vis-à-vis* wider socio-cultural issues.

Nelson's chapter (Chapter 11) suggests that attention to the 'small things' that nurses have used and made over time, rather than to the grand narratives of nursing's history, can illuminate both the socio-political context of nursing practice as well as nurses' accomplishments. Nelson begins by offering a critique of historical approaches to the analysis of nursing practice that focus on issues of truth and constructivism, and discusses emergent trends in critical histories that illuminate the relationships between social practice, technologies and power. She shows how a 'history of the present' approach to investigation highlights the historically contingent and partial nature of social change. She stresses the importance of histories that contrast with the evolutionary and triumphant tone of conventional, 'subject-centred' nursing history. History, used as political tool for promoting nursing, has been developed and legitimised by nurses through its association with a positive tradition whose aim is to establish the facts and eradicate bias. The difficulty, Nelson argues, is that these approaches desocialise nursing history and erase not just nursing's intractable problems, but also the social and political issues which mediate how nursing has been practised, defined and understood.

Nelson explicates a method for a critical history which focuses on the materiality of nurses' practices, including the specificities of nurses' written records, procedure manuals and the everyday items of nursing practice, such as implements and dressings. Through attention to these materials and the practices which employ their use, Nelson gives a compelling account of how the significance of local factors (such as available technology), and broad contextual issues (such as gender and religion), can be surfaced in the emergence, proliferation and demise of nursing practices.

In the last and concluding chapter, I offer an account of my own approach to researching. This approach recognises that nurses are embedded in relations, but that there is not one, but many 'others' to whom they relate. My work has therefore been at pains to stress how nurses perform to multiple agendas, multiple others. Thus the chapter offers an approach which draws together particular ethnographic and analytic methods in ways that help us to 'get inside' nurses' relations to show that they constitute much more than a patient–nurse dyad. Specifically, I discuss why researchers should travel to the bedside and track patients through all aspects of nursing work and hospital life. I show why patients need to be understood both as persons and as the virtual object figured through nurses' and others representations of them.

References

Benner, P. (1984) *From Novice to Expert: Excellence and Power in Clinical Nursing Practice*. Menlo Park, CA: Addison-Wesley.

Fernandez, J.W. (1986) *Persuasions and Performances. The Play of Tropes in Culture*. Bloomington, IN: Indiana University Press.

Giddens, A. (1991) *Modernity and Self-identity: Self and Society in the Late Modern Age*. Cambridge: Polity Press.

Lyotard, J.F. (1984) *The Post-modern Condition: A Report on Knowledge*. Manchester: Manchester University Press.

Rudge, T. (1997) *Nursing wounds: a discourse analysis of nurse–patient interactions during wound care procedures in a burns unit*. PhD dissertation, La Trobe University, Australia.

Silverman, D. (1989) Six rules of qualitative research: a post-romantic argument. *Symbolic Interaction* **12**: 215–30.

Silverman, D. and Gubrium, J. (1989) Introduction. In D. Silverman and J. Gubrium (eds) *The Politics of Field Research: Sociology beyond Enlightenment*. London: Sage, pp. 1–12.

PART I

Fields

In this part, May and Purkis explore what the notion of dynamic practice means for the idea of researching a field. Qualitative methodologies usually engage researchers in fieldwork. This term suggests that qualitative research is concerned with 'naturally' occurring events and practices, rather than those which are determined by the research, through either a laboratory or other kind of experiment. What is important here is not just that a field of practice is a place people have feelings about; rather, the idea of a field helps to remind us that it is *experienced* in very particular and specific ways. In this way the idea of studying a field of practice helps remind us that it is a *lived* space.

However, the term 'field' can also be deceptive: it suggests that the field is a given, a bounded space, which can be entered and observed. In contrast, a politically sensitive approach acknowledges that the field is itself a construct, a 'site' (cf. Turner, 1989). But critical to the way in which the field is approached is the question, what or who is doing the constructing? For example, the way the researcher 'enters' the field prefigures the field in ways which affect the researcher's capacity to 'represent' (Coffey and Atkinson, 1995) or evoke (Tyler, 1986) it. Consequently, how a field researcher answers the question, who or what is constructing the field, depends upon their methodology.

For example, our approach to the field can acknowledge that, yes, the field is lived, but the parameters that define and dissect the field lie outside the power and control of those living it. Here the field is understood as a function or effect of social structures, such as dominant gender or class relations. Here a researcher may enter the field to 'get' accounts of subjects' experiences of the field, or to find out more about what they do, in terms of restraint, values and norms, for example. Researchers in this methodological tradition, while acknowledging that the field is lived, enter it as if it is *pre-constructed*. The difficulty here is that the subjects of field research may end up appearing like 'cultural dopes' (Garfinkel, 1967), at the mercy of those structures that define the field, so that their creativity as *social beings* is effaced.

How can we get a balance? We can understand the idea of a field differently. First, with contemporary anthropologists, such as Geertz (1993), we can understand that there is not one field, but many potential fields, which are constituted by the researched as they interact in the course of their daily lives. Second, we can also understand that these actors, as they go about their daily lives are not free agents. So we can seek ways to make explicit how socio-cultural relations position research subjects as at the same time they are themselves active participants in those relations. Third, we can, with the post-structuralists, understand that the field is made up of different and sometimes competing representations: that there is not one field which means the same to everyone, but multiple possible meanings and interests. If we take this approach to the field we must pay attention to power effects and how they are accomplished.

References

Coffey, A. and Atkinson, P. (1995) *Making Sense of Qualitative Data*. London: Sage.

Garfinkel, H. (1967) *Studies in Ethnomethodology*. Englewood Cliffs, NJ: Prentice Hall.

Geertz, C. (1993) *The Interpretation of Cultures*. London: Fontana.

Turner, R. (1989) Deconstructing the field. In D. Silverman and J. Gubrium (eds) *The Politics of Field Research: Sociology beyond Enlightenment*. London: Sage, pp. 13–29.

Tyler, S.A. (1986) Post-modern ethnography: from document of the occult to occult document. In J. Clifford and G. Marcus (eds) *Writing Culture: The Poetics and Politics of Ethnography*. Berkeley: California University Press.

CHAPTER 2

Where do we stand in relation to the data? Being reflexive about reflexivity in health care evaluation

Carl May

This book stems from the recognition that while there are many texts for nurses that focus upon the practice of qualitative inquiry, the majority of these are about the application of specific techniques. However, there are far fewer that address problems of theory and reflexivity – the very things from which qualitative inquiry draws its analytic and explanatory strength – and these are the very focus of this book.

My purpose in this chapter is to address some considerations of reflexivity in qualitative inquiry from the perspective of evaluation research (ER). ER is important because it is one domain of research that increasingly employs qualitative techniques to develop an understanding of policy and practice in health care. It is therefore one of the key approaches to health services research. Within that community of practice, qualitative approaches to ER are undercut by the elision of theory, and so the question of reflexivity is undercut by the circumstances and objectives of the kinds of question and research problem on which evaluation researchers focus.

Because I am interested in how 'theory' can be drawn into the foreground in debates about ER, I want to address problems of power and subjectivity in this chapter. These issues raise complex epistemological and ontological problems in ER, but are rarely considered in an explicit way in the debates around method and practice in this field of research activity. My point of departure is a broadly constructionist one, where the social relations (and the social spaces) around which ER is oriented are understood to be problematic.

The chapter is structured around four broad topics. First, I address the vexed place of social theory within ER. Second, I am concerned with how data collection is substantively different in ER from some other arenas of research. Third, I explore the problem of reflexivity for the researcher in ER contexts. Finally, I draw some conclusions about the problem of power and subjectivity in such research. In constructing the chapter in this way I am concerned with exploring the social organisation of professional knowledge and practice, and the ways that these shape and are shaped by new health technologies, modalities of treatment, and configurations of service organisation and delivery. As a sociologist and as an eva-luation researcher these are the questions that I address in my everyday research practice: but I recognise that I address them in different ways according to normative expectations that are poli-tically, as well as methodologically, shaped. What follows is therefore a critique of some of the ways that qualitative inquiry is deployed within ER.

What is ER and why is it a problem?

Many researchers whose work deploys the theories and methods of qualitative inquiry do so from a position that favours highly theorised (and frequently abstract) perspectives on the nature of social phenomena and on the practices through which these are understood (Johnson, 1999). Yet other researchers take an approach to qualitative inquiry that treats the role and place of theory as *unproblematic*. This kind of approach is one that is dominated by concrete questions about policy and practice that are about the operational efficacy and utility of particular configura-tions of service organisation and delivery, or about the improve-ment of treatments and services. This emphasis fits well with the thrust towards evidence-based services that has been a crucial feature of policy debates about the organisation of public services of all kinds, and of health care in particular (Harrison, 1996, 1999). An equally important domain of such research, that impacts steadily and heavily on providers and recipients of health care, is the constant push towards evaluation. ER is directed at this kind of problem, and the place for qualitative inquiry within it has been set out precisely on the grounds that it can deliver answers to some of these key questions. For example, in their introduction to qualitative methods for clinicians, Pope and Mays (2001: 77) assert that:

'Health Services Research has become more prominent as a result of the NHS reforms. Both providers and purchasers want to know exactly where the money is spent, and how it could be used more effectively. How best to obtain information about health services is the subject of some debate within and between disciplines engaged in such research ... For effective research both quantitative and qualitative approaches need to be used.'

In other words, qualitative inquiry is one component of a wider battery of methods that can be employed to answer evaluative questions about effectiveness, utility, and most of all, value for money. In this context, one of the key criticisms of ER has been that it seems to be an *atheoretical* field of research work, that is primarily about assessing particular kinds of services and treatment modalities. Elsewhere, David Pilgrim and I have observed that

'Social scientists who are employed to conduct health service research ... in the British National Health Service are subjected to two forms of constraint or influence upon their disciplinary identity... The first of these relates to the power of their employers to define research questions, shape methodology and control the dissemination of research findings... [The second is that] the nature of applied research is changing. In particular it is being constituted by temporary, multidisciplinary arrangements which are problem focused. This renders unidisciplinary knowledge vulnerable.' (Pilgrim & May, 1998: 43)

What this can mean is that practitioners of ER practise in conditions where theory is subordinated to answering specific kinds of concrete question defined by policy relevance. In this context, researchers in the field increasingly pursue three kinds of problem (May & Purkis, 1997):

1. The division of labour in health care has become increasingly complex, and is characterised by changes in the organisation of

local authority and responsibility. Generic managers contest clinicians' control over professional activities, treatment decisions, resource allocation and cost control.

2. The rapid growth of consumerism has involved the notion that service users are well equipped to adjudicate over the quality of treatment decisions and the quality of professional care that they receive. This has led to demands for users' views about services to be collected and disseminated.

3. Purchasers of health services demand information to guide their decision making. They seek data about operational and cost effectiveness, as well as about alternative methods of service delivery.

The demand for evaluative research, and for rapid appraisal, which has dominated health care provision in the UK over the past decade, has created an increasing range of opportunities for social science researchers of all kinds. Equally, researchers from within the clinical professions have chosen to adopt modes of social inquiry from within the social sciences. The effect of this is that the boundaries between pure and applied research are increasingly blurred and permeable; it also means that the way that data is constructed and interpreted is defined in relation to a variety of political conditions and considerations. It is important not to overplay the place of theory in the wider arena of research: much empirical research that deploys the methods and philosophical positions of qualitative inquiry often does so on the basis of exaggerated allegiances to specific theoretical perspectives (Johnson, 1999).

However much ER is criticised for its apparently atheoretical approach to research problems, and for its concreteness – around, for example, evaluating particular service configurations, or assessing new health technologies – this cannot mean that the researcher is immune to the kinds of epistemological and methodological problem that are encountered in other domains of social inquiry. Quite the reverse is true, although there seems to be little opportunity within the field of ER to interrogate these difficulties more closely. The tendency is therefore to systematically exclude deep questions about the status of research practice and its products from discussion about the conduct and outcomes of such work

(May *et al.*, 2000), and to locate these in other arenas of debate. The question that this chapter raises, about where the researcher stands *in relation to the data*, is difficult to centrally deploy in ER yet remains of central importance to the conduct of such work. This is especially so given the push towards including different kinds of qualitative inquiry within its domain.

In summary, evaluation research is a problem for practitioners of qualitative inquiry because of its focus on concrete questions of policy and practice, and because the apparent abstraction of inductive research techniques is difficult to square with the political demand to produce the answer to those concrete questions in a way that meets the normative expectations of ER's sponsors. From this stems a further, deeper problem, which is the shifting status of the research act, and of the interpretation of data, in such circumstances. While the specific techniques employed in this kind of work may be those recommended in a wider literature about interrogating and understanding the phenomenology of subjective experience, its effects *in* practice, and *on* practices, may be rather different.

Qualitative inquiry is substantively different in specific ER settings

The identity of the researcher is at the heart of the reflexivity question in qualitative inquiry, and is a long-standing source of debate – especially amongst feminist researchers who have either assumed or sought common cause with the subjects of their research. Ann Oakley (Oakley, 1981) has been a leading proponent of the view that the boundaries between researcher and researched are politically shaped, and that they can thus be *reshaped* according to the shared experiences of participants. The effect of this debate has been to problematise the construction of the researcher as insider/outsider, and to suggest the emancipatory potential of qualitative inquiry as a means of giving voice to groups of respondents. The background to this is the notion that respondents are often disempowered by the institutional structures in which they are located. These structures range from macro-level patterns of social organisation (e.g. the social organisation of gendered work) to their micro-level exemplars (e.g. patterns of gendered work and their implication in specific practices at the level of the hospital ward). Through qualitative methods, it has been argued, the deep experiences and views of the researched are drawn safely into the public sphere in ways that permit them to be heard, and perhaps to influence policy. One area in which this view has evinced tremendous resonance has been in the field of health care practice around people with HIV/AIDS (Crossley, 1998).

It is in this context that qualitative inquiry has come to be seen, as Kath Melia has observed (Melia, 1981), as a means by which individuals and groups can 'tell it like it is'. Her now famous study of the occupational socialisation of student nurses has come to be seen as an exemplar of this approach. There are, however, multiple ways of 'telling it like it is', and Melia has recently come to reflect on the 'adequacy of interview data' in explaining the social world of the student nurses that she interviewed in her study. In particular, she is concerned about the status of the interview as a handle on the social world of the respondent.

> 'Informal interview data are yielded by a series of questions and general lines of enquiry embedded in a seemingly natural conversation with the interviewee. The data can be seen, then, as an account of the interviewee's opinions and views arrived at as a result of interaction with the researcher. The effect of this interaction cannot be denied.' (Melia, 1997: 34)

In evaluation research, the effect of this interaction needs to be assessed, not simply as the product of processes of intersubjectivity and construction, but also as the product of institutional processes of adjudication and surveillance. My point here is a simple one: that respondents or subjects in ER studies are confronted with a relationship characterised by knowledge seeking on behalf of agencies that often intend to shape and reshape key constituents of their social world, most obviously their experience of work. The reflexivity of the researcher, therefore, is that of an agent of a set of power/knowledge relations that penetrates and reshapes attempts to share experiences and meanings. The insider/outsider boundary, so important across the arena of social science research practice, is not blurred here, but instead is drawn into sharp relief. Interviews that I undertake as an evaluation researcher go towards understanding the 'quality' of a particular set of professional practices, or of configurations of knowledge, through constructing a view of the effectiveness of professionals' practice by which they might be judged.

This element of judgement that sits within the conduct of qualitative inquiry as a component of ER is one that sits uncomfortably in the wider frame of discourse about qualitative research. It raises awkward questions about the notion of giving voice, and about the immediate circumstances of the interaction between researcher and researched. Most importantly, it manifests the power relations that are inherent in the encounter (whether formed around interview or around observation). In this context, the very concreteness and immediacy of ER questions (Does this service work? Do patients like it? Is it cost effective?) renders ever more troubling the question 'where do we stand in relation to the data?'

Reflexivity and qualitative inquiry: power and surveillance

So far, I have made two key points. The first is that the domain of ER is one where research questions are concrete and immediate in their form, and are predicated on the notion that research is intended to engender change in the configuration and organisation of health care. The second is that, within ER, the business of conducting qualitative inquiry does not always sit well with an inductive approach that privileges the voice(s) of subject groups – who might sometimes themselves be powerful in influencing the kinds of question that are asked in ER. Because these are such important elements of the business of qualitative inquiry, I want now to turn to the problem of power.

Qualitative inquiry in ER settings is about the intricate linkages between power and knowledge. In circumstances where what is at issue is the construction of management information, the kind of power/knowledge bundling that we find suggested in the writings of Michel Foucault is quite literally *real*. Here, Foucault asserts that power is expressed in the business of governance:

'The exercise of power consists in guiding the possibility of conduct and putting in order the possible outcomes. Basically, power is less of a confrontation between two adversaries or the linking of one to another than a question of government. This word must be allowed the very broad meaning that it had in the 16th century. "Government" did not refer to political structures or to the management of states; rather it designated the way in which the conduct of individuals might be directed... To govern in this sense is to structure the possible field of action for others.' (Foucault, 1986: 221)

In the intersubjective organisation of 'being known' and 'knowing', then, power is constituted and experienced. Indeed, the business of *knowing* is one to which the different institutions that characterise late modernity have invested an enormous degree of effort. The practices through which this is constituted operate through the kinds of 'gaze' that Foucault suggests form the ways that knowledge is conceived of and produced in health care – for example, in a shift from knowledge about objects as the focus of clinical practice and procedure to knowledge about the experience of subjects – as well as the kinds of knowledge that are generated in ER. Foucault has written at length about the role of the human sciences (psychology, psychiatry, sociology and statistics) in constituting and sustaining particular ways of thinking about the subject (Foucault, 1973, 1977; Barker, 1998), and in doing so constituting identities and communities of practice. Discourse, Foucault reminds us, constitutes its own objects (Foucault, 1986).

The application of qualitative inquiry to ER, then, forms an arena where power is mobilised and experiences are transformed. Qualitative inquiry more generally is about 'giving voice' to subjective experiences through intersubjective processes, and thus constituting a particular 'truth' about the meanings and practices through which these subjective experiences are formed. In ER, qualitative inquiry is quite simply one of a number of modes of surveillance exercised over subjects – what Lasch (1979), in another context, has called the 'social invasion of the self' – and which is intended to penetrate the private and authentic concerns (feelings, anxieties, worries and so forth) of particular actors. It is important not to overplay the notion that power is exercised within the constitution of knowledge in qualitative inquiry, for although it undoubtedly is exercised, there are degrees of knowledge and so degrees of power. But one way to see the role of qualitative inquiry in ER is to draw a direct parallel with the notion that health professionals are increasingly expected to 'know' their patients as more than simply representatives of a particular disease or disability, that is, as specific instances of a pathology. Instead, there is a kind of power exemplified in the shift to 'holistim' that

> 'finds its expression in a therapeutic gaze directed at the production of truth about the subject. Through being "known" and through "talking and listening" the patient is encouraged to give voice to private and authentic concerns – and so to produce her own truth... In this sense, there is not only a direct and intimate connection between "work" and "relationships", but for all practical purposes the two are indivisible.' (May, 1992: 597–8)

For the purposes of the present chapter, we could replace the word 'patient' with 'interviewee' to good effect. What I am getting at here is the sense in which qualitative inquiry involves an encounter that has a confessional quality. The conventional promise to respondents that interview data will be in some way anonymised is as much an implicit recognition of this as it is an explicit 'ethical' constraint. It evinces the connections between a range of practices and their effects. The problematisation of the subject in the human sciences (and of the specific construction of the subject in qualitative inquiry within them) has led to the organisation of institutional practices that harness and co-opt interior knowledge about subjects, and which deploy these in ways that, intentionally or not, extends corporate control over them.

It is important not to construe the position that I have adopted here as an excessively bleak or nihilistic one, but it is equally important to understand that it expresses some of the *Realpolitik* of qualitative inquiry in ER settings. Qualitative inquiry can never be politically neutral, and in work that is directed at 'understanding' the social organisation of health care practice it does contribute to the shaping and reshaping of institutional patterns of practice themselves. An outstanding example of this is the impact of Glaser and Strauss's work on the social organisation of terminal care, which has exercised the most profound effect, directly and indirectly, on the care of the dying since its publication in 1965 (Glaser & Strauss, 1965). Qualitative inquiry does this precisely because its methodological strategy is often to *individualise* subjects. Respondents in such studies cannot escape an awareness of this, and an awareness that what they say has consequences that extend a good deal beyond the interactional setting of the interview into an arena where individualisation is predicated on opening up the subjective interior. Dreyfus and Rabinow have argued that

> 'The conviction that truth can be examined through the self-examination of consciousness and the confession of one's thoughts and acts now appears so natural, so compelling, indeed so self-evident, that it seems unreasonable to posit that such a self-examination is a central component in a strategy of power. This unseemliness rests on our attachment to the repressive hypothesis; if the truth is inherently opposed to power, then its uncovering would surely lead us on the path to liberation.' (Dreyfus & Rabinow, 1986: 175)

This kind of perspective runs through qualitative inquiry, as much as it does the massive shift towards subjectification (Giddens, 1991) that is such a profound feature of late modernity. The point here is that qualitative research in ER is not just the crude application of a system of practices by which knowledge and power are interwoven in specific corporate settings. Rather, it must be seen against the background of the construction of subjects and subjectivities that are effected by 'research' itself, across the human sciences. ER can therefore be seen as a particular, highly focused and applied set of primarily evaluative practices located within that wider set of configurations.

Being reflexive about power in qualitative inquiry, then, is vital because the question, 'where do we stand in relation to the data?' needs to be assessed by reference to our own place as researchers in a much broader configuration of knowledge production, and our identity as agents of particular kinds of power/knowledge. Our shared experiences might not necessarily be those that we suppose them to be.

In her wonderful book *The History of the Modern Fact*, Mary Poovey (1998) shows how the very idea of quantitative *data* depended upon the invention of rhetorical strategies that neutralised the political or moral content of knowledge. This is a consistent theme of critical studies of the history of quantification in social inquiry (Porter, 1986, 1995). For practitioners of *qualitative* inquiry, the notion of neutrality is anathema. Qualitative data is imbued with social, political and cultural meanings and cannot be otherwise (Coffey & Atkinson, 1996). It can be read in multiple ways (Atkinson, 1990), and within its frame it is impossible to claim a linear set of truths about the practices that it draws into view (May & Ellis, 2001). All of this presents particular kinds of problems in the set of practices that are interlinked to form the 'field' of evaluation research.

Given the grimly unreflexive nature of some of the literature that prescribes the procedures and techniques by which evaluation may be accomplished using qualitative techniques, we should perhaps not be too surprised that these problems are systematically represented across the ER literature. The emergence of a 'how to do it' literature that privileges explicit procedures for data collection and collation over the analytic and interpretive practices, had led to suggestions of a 'drift to positivism' within qualitative inquiry more generally (Johnson, 1999).

How can we get past all of this, and stand in relation to the data in a more satisfactory and productive way. First of all, within the practices of qualitative inquiry – however these are formulated – particular kinds of social space are being opened for dialogue and engagement. One methods text places this at the centre of its account of technique:

> 'Qualitative research is part of debate, not fixed truth. Qualitative research is (a) an attempt to capture the sense that lies within, that structures what we say and what we do; (b) an exploration, elaborating the significance of a defined phenomena; (c) the illuminative representation of the meaning of a delimited issue or problem.' (Banister *et al.*, 1994: 3)

This is actually about finding a way into, and through, the diffuse discourse of the *social* (Turner, 1995) that is constituted through the application of the human sciences to the production of what Foucault has called 'technologies of the self' (Foucault, 1977). That is, it is about the production and representation of selves through the production of narrative (May & Fleming, 1997). If all of this seems a bit far from the pragmatic business of assessing whether a service is effective or not, it is important to remember that there is no 'service' without subjects.

Second, the incorporation of qualitative inquiry within ER constitutes particular objects of practice. That is to say, however methods are expected to engender the production of subjective 'truths', their organisation in practice often systematically excludes those that are not constituted through the rhetoric of corporate ambition. Understanding the effectiveness of a service, or the utility of a treatment intervention, cannot always be run through with other kinds of truth – perhaps politically inconvenient ones about resistance and transformation. Indeed, where it is, it becomes difficult to present an evaluation in ways that actually meet the demands of a sponsoring agency. If we engage with Foucault's dictum, that 'discourse constitutes its own objects', then we must recognise that this is a dictum that defines not just productive spheres of inclusion, but also what is *not to be known or understood*.

Concluding comment

Of course, there are many different kinds of evaluation research, and the sorts of problem that I have discussed in this chapter vary in the extent to which they affect its conduct. However, I have outlined three kinds of problem that both *affect* the conduct of qualitative inquiry in ER, and thus *effect* its products:

1. Evaluation research (ER) is too frequently assumed to be the product of the neutral application of self-evident research techniques.
2. The application of techniques of qualitative inquiry within ER can subvert attempts to 'give voice' to respondents, in favour of practices of adjudication.
3. Qualitative inquiry within ER can co-opt and mobilise subjectivity in ways that can extend corporate control through practices of surveillance.

The principal point that needs to be made here is that these are not simply isolated problems, but actually form the key feature of a process by which evaluation research is politicised. It is crucial to keep the political nature of evaluation research in sight, for 'evidence' is increasingly *the* device through which political disputes around the organisation of health care are framed. It might even be that the social production of evidence *is* the politics of health care.

This has important implications for the evaluative researcher, who becomes in this context a political actor. So, one, very important, answer to the question 'where do we stand in relation to the data?' must be that our relation to it is one of concrete political significance. When the evaluation researcher deploys the techniques (and analytic positions) of qualitative inquiry it is to effect a contribution to a political process, and to intervene in the production of evidence. No one can be neutral in such a process, and claims that are made about the data and its analytic products in ER need to be run through with ontological, as well as epistemological caution.

Acknowledgements

As ever, I am grateful to Christine May for her critical reading of my work, and to Joanna Latimer for invaluable editorial comments.

References

Atkinson, P. (1990) *The Ethnographic Imagination: Textual Constructions of Reality*. London: Routledge.

Banister, P., Burman, E., Parker, I., Taylor, M. & Tindall, C. (1994) *Qualitative Methods in Psychology: A Research Guide*. Buckingham: Open University Press.

Barker, P. (1998) *Michel Foucault: An Introduction*. Edinburgh: Edinburgh University Press.

Coffey, A. & Atkinson, P. (1996) *Making Sense of Qualitative Data*. London: Sage.

Crossley, M. (1998) 'Sick role' or 'empowerment'? The ambiguities of life with an HIV positive diagnosis. *Sociology of Health & Illness* 20: 507–31.

Dreyfus, H.L. & Rabinow, P. (1986) *Michel Foucault: Beyond Structuralism and Hermeneutics*. Brighton: Harvester.

Foucault, M. (1973) *The Birth of the Clinic*. London: Tavistock.

Foucault, M. (1977) *Discipline and Punish: The Birth of the Prison*. Harmondsworth: Penguin.

Foucault, M. (1986) Afterword: the subject and power. In H.L. Dreyfus &

P. Rabinow (eds) *Michel Foucalt: Beyond Structuralism and Hermeneutics*. Brighton: Harvester, pp. 208–26.

Giddens, A. (1991) *Modernity and Self-identity: Self and Society in the Late Modern Age*. Cambridge: Polity Press.

Glaser, B.G. & Strauss, A. (1965) *Awareness of Dying*. Chicago: Aldine.

Harrison, S. (1996) The politics of evidence-based medicine in the United Kingdom. *Policy and Politics* **26**: 15–31.

Harrison, S. (1999) Clinical autonomy and health policy: past and futures. In M. Exworthy & S. Halford (eds) *Professionals and the New Managerialism in the Public Sector*. Buckingham: Open University Press, pp. 50–64.

Johnson, M. (1999) Observations on science and pseudoscience in nursing research. *Journal of Advanced Nursing* **30**: 67–73.

Lasch, C. (1979) *The Culture of Narcissism*. New York: W.W. Norton.

May, C. (1992) Individual care? Power and subjectivity in therapeutic relationships. *Sociology* **26**: 589–602.

May, C. & Ellis, N.T. (2001) When protocols fail: technical evaluation, biomedical knowledge, and the social construction of facts about a telemedicine clinic. *Social Science and Medicine* **53**: 989–1002.

May, C. & Fleming, C. (1997) The professional imagination: narrative and the symbolic boundaries between medicine and nursing. *Journal of Advanced Nursing* **25**: 1094–1100.

May, C. & Purkis, M.E. (1997) Professional power and professional relations. *Health and Social Care in the Community* **5**: 1–3.

May, C., Mort, M., Mair, F., Ellis, N.T. & Gask, L. (2000) Evaluation of new technologies in health care systems: what's the context?, *Health Informatics Journal* **6**: 64–8.

Melia, K. (1981) Student nurses' accounts of their work and training: a qualitative analysis. PhD dissertation, University of Edinburgh.

Melia, K. (1997) Producing plausible stories: interviewing student nurses. In G. Miller & R. Dingwall (eds) *Context and Method in Qualitative Research*. London: Sage, pp. 26–36.

Oakley, A. (1981) Interviewing women: a contradiction in terms. In H. Roberts (ed.) *Doing Feminist Research*. London: Routledge & Kegan Paul.

Pilgrim, D. & May, C. (1998) Social scientists and the British National Health Service. *Social Science and Health* **4**: 42–54.

Poovey, M. (1998) *A History of the Modern Fact: Problems of Knowledge in the Sciences of Wealth and Society*. Chicago: University of Chicago Press.

Pope, C. & Mays, N. (2001) Opening the black box: an encounter in the corridors of health services research. In N. Mays & C. Pope (eds) *Qualitative Research in Health Care*. London: BMJ Publications, pp. 68–76.

Porter, T.M. (1986) *The Rise of Statistical Thinking, 1820–1900*. Princeton, NJ: Princeton University Press.

Porter, T.M. (1995) *Trust in Numbers: The Pursuit of Objectivity in Science and Public Life*. Princeton, NJ: Princeton University Press.

Turner, B.S. (1995) *Medical Power and Social Knowledge*, 2nd edn. London: Sage.

CHAPTER 3

Moving nursing practice: integrating theory and method

Mary Ellen Purkis

A field in motion

Field studies represent a relatively low-technology, low-cost method for studying dynamic processes that result in an accomplishment we call 'nursing practice.' On the face of it, all that is required is a reasonably discreet observer, someone who has a keen eye for detail, a capacity to recall events, to write those down as soon as possible after they have occurred. Someone with a reasonable sense of curiosity who can engage people in conversations about their everyday activities. So it is interesting that there are few such studies to be found within nursing's vast research literature. Where 'interpretative' studies of nursing practice are undertaken, researchers have more often turned to grounded theory – perhaps because a standard approach has been established (Glaser & Strauss, 1967; Strauss & Corbin, 1997); the path is clearer. It is this apparent clarity associated with the conduct of grounded theory that draws researchers in. For, while the gathering of materials for the conduct of a field study is relatively straightforward, the interpretation of that material is anything but. Once all the material has been transcribed and has been sorted into neat piles, the researcher is left facing the question, 'what does it all mean?' The choices about how to make it all mean something are rarely, if ever, evident. One 'choice' that has been successful for myself and for many of my graduate students is to simply begin reading. Reading nursing, reading social theory, reading philosophy, reading transcripts. Reading until questions begin to form and you find those questions repeatedly on scraps of paper and in the margins of what you have been reading.

The questions that I often return to revolve around the paradox of the singularity and uniqueness of individual nurse–patient encounters against the remarkable standardization of practice across encounters. What follows is an examination (one in a long series!) of how nursing practice can be *made standard* within the context of a field study of nursing practice. I also illustrate how practice can be presented as a momentary and unique accomplishment by drawing on different theoretical traditions, different questions, and different representations of practice.

Health promotion: a mission for nursing

One of the most pronounced obsessions for professional nursing over the past century has been that of establishing itself as a legitimate, autonomous discipline, distinct from medicine and its concern for the diseased body and distinct from social work and its concern for the mind and soul of societal members. With the advent of a discourse of 'health promotion' in the late 1960s and early 1970s, it seemed that the profession's identity problems were solved. Over the past 30 years or so, nurse theorists have been busy developing a theoretical space which nursing could occupy and call its own. These theoretical developments have been organized conceptually such that 'health' must be described as the foci of nursing's gaze (Fawcett, 1995) and that the promotion of health becomes the force driving the calculation of nursing outcomes (Gottlieb, 1981; AARN, 1987; Pender, 1987; Meleis, 1990; Stewart, 1995; Lindsey & Hartrick, 1996; Liepert, 1999; O'Brien-Pallas & Baumann, 2000).

The domain of health promotion is not, however, an uncontested one. Nutritionists claim it. Physiotherapists claim it. Occupational therapists claim it. Psychotherapists claim it. Alternative health practitioners claim it. Even city planners claim it (Petersen & Lupton, 1996). And, interestingly, medicine has, over the past few years, shown increasingly that it too wishes to lay claim to this domain of practice.

And so, this is one part of the problem facing nursing to the extent it conceives itself as a practice discipline: having 'discovered' a domain of practice to call its own, it enters that domain to find it already occupied and with others banging down the door trying to get in. What any good marketer would do at this point is say, 'Ah! But our brand of X is better than that of our competitors! Try it, you'll like ours better!' This strategy is not as callous as it may appear. As health professionals, we are constantly bombarded with 'market' rhetoric and it is not surprising that we should pick up on this discourse within which our practices are increasingly being positioned (de la Cuesta, 1994). Indeed, nurses in the field setting to be explored more fully in this chapter were observed to compare their health messages as of better quality than those of family members and general medical practitioners (Purkis, 2001). And so, within the rhetoric of a market economy, nurses in practice have been busy positioning themselves as the bearers of high quality, legitimate health knowledge that is beneficial to people of all ages. And, on the basis of fieldwork conducted in a number of settings over the past decade, they can be said to be quite effective within this domain.

I want to make a distinction here between nurses in practice and those who write about nursing practice, because within that latter group often the reverse story is told. Nurses are said to be reluctant to move away from a 'medical model of practice'. They are said to be failing to adequately represent their practice and its health promoting effects (Anderson *et al.*, 1994). These discrepant understandings about practice have fascinated me for many years now. Can it be that the writers simply do not understand practice? This is not an unfamiliar position for practitioners to take in relation to academic nurses. Or, are practitioners misguided about what it is they are doing in practice: this position represents a vast majority of the theoretical literature within nursing.

I will adopt a middle position on these views. It is my contention that those who seek to theorize nursing practice have made use of conceptual tools inadequate to the task upon which they are embarking. It is also my contention that, in the intensity of engaging in the important work of accomplishing one's identity as a nurse in everyday encounters with patients, practitioners are not well positioned to view themselves and their actions critically. Nor should this be a strongly advocated position as it instantiates a form of social distancing (Vollstedt, 1999) that does not always serve the interests of those patients. This is not to say that nursing practice requires no 'improvement'. It does mean, however, that I do not intend, in this chapter, to put myself in a position to *prescribe* the direction of that improvement. I believe nurses in practice themselves are likely best positioned to take up from my argument the directions they wish to follow in the interests of high-quality patient care.

The argument that will be advanced is one that maintains nursing practice in positive regard: that is, it establishes itself on a ground where nurses are understood to be knowledgeable actors working dynamically to accomplish their practice – whatever they may take that to be. And, within a context where nurses take 'health promotion' to be the goal of their practice, the argument I make is that nurses 'know' that the promotion of health is too narrow a practice domain for nursing to operate within. Nurses have become 'expert' at translating their care of patients' bodies into the language of health promotion, and in so doing they may be accomplishing a radical separation of their talk about practice from their primary access to practice: the body of the patient. Such a radical separation requires critical attention if nursing is to remain a productive sphere of activity within contemporary health care delivery. Research methodologies are needed that can conceptualize nursing as an active and knowledgeable social accomplishment. The accounts of nursing that these methodologies produce can then be held against the reporting of nursing practice. Only then can the radical separation between what nurses take to be their work and the actual work they are accomplishing be made explicit as an effect of organizational imperatives that influence the ways in which nursing care is reported.

This argument will be explored in more depth within the next three sections. First, I will explore this issue of 'inadequate conceptual tools' for the task of explicating nursing as a dynamic social accomplishment. Second, I will explore an example of nursing practice in which the nurse and the mother whom she is counselling are both seen to be engrossed (Goffman, 1974) in the accomplishment of their mutual identities. The plasticity of identity is explored in terms of Fernandez' notion of 'persuasion and performance' (Fernandez, 1986). Specifically, the encounter between the nurse and the mother is analysed as a form of *argumentation*. What is at stake is the identity of each protagonist and their authority to determine what is (or what is not) *healthy*. Nursing practice in this approach appears dynamic, and identity, like health promotion, emerges not as given, prescribed by fixed and stable categories, but as accomplished. The chapter concludes with discussion about how nursing has placed the practices of health promotion within its boundaries, and how the spaces for critique offered within this placement leave little room for examining nursing as a powerful influence within what is treated as a power-neutral set of practices.

Nursing: a practice discipline

Having entered into the business of constructing itself as an academic discipline rather recently in comparison with the more established professions of medicine and law, nurses have not been slow in developing theoretical models that they claim *guide* practice. These models are said to support and legitimate the movement of nursing out of the realm of lay caring and later hospital 'training' into the academy proper. Yet, if this is their purpose, to guide practice of an intellectually advanced sort, these models are rather curious things. For the most part they prescribe for nurses ways of dividing up persons as particular sorts of entity who are already, or can become, susceptible to nursing care.[1] To exemplify the point, it has become a commonplace within the theoretical literature to identify patients as 'bio-psycho-social-spiritual beings' (Roy, 1984). The implication for the practitioner is that each of these segments of the patient is to be investigated for malfunction. The appropriate action taken to promote health in one or more of these spheres then stands as the 'outcome' of nursing care. These theoretical models, in effect, represent information processing, problem-solving strategies that nurses are encouraged to take up in order to legitimate and justify the expenditures made on them by financially strapped health care organizations.

Such segmenting of patients, however, 'pre-figures' (Strathern, 1991) the discipline of nursing for enrolment into new management technologies now extending their reach throughout organized health services worldwide. For instance, Latimer (1995: 216) argues that

'In associating themselves with particular devices such as information processing, problem-solving models of action, there may be particular effects upon the possibilities for how nurses can think, say or do as they practice. Thus, in enrolling particular managerial devices, nurses themselves may be enlisted in managerial programmes in unexpected ways.'

So, rather than 'guiding' the practice of autonomous health care professionals, the argument advanced here is that these models have extended the reach and effect of managerialist interests in predicting and controlling health care costs.

A further problem with these theoretical constructions of the practice discipline of nursing is that they imply a static (Elias & Kilminster, 1991) relationship between the nurse and the patient. The extolled necessity is that all patients be 'assessed' because each one will exhibit different features of their individualized bio-psycho-social-spiritual selves. However, what is not questioned is that the proper focus of the nurse will be on the person *as* a bio-psycho-social-spiritual being and that the person opens him or herself up to the nurse *as* such a being. That is, people are being treated within these theoretical constructions as already set and fully accomplished as 'nurses' and 'patients'. There is no sense of movement in and out of these organizing positions. There is no sense that the terrain of health promotion is contested. As such, there can be no recognition – on the part of the nurse or of the patient – of resistance to being in a particular position, *to being positioned*.

Promoting health as a settled practice

An example may help to illustrate the difficulties I am alluding to here. In a field study of community nursing practice in Canada, Peggy-Anne Field (1989) writes in the following manner about the practice as she claims to have 'observed' it:

'Another client, Charles, *chose* not to take his pills (for tuberculosis) because he *knew* drinking and drugs were con-traindicated. *Because he made a conscious decision*, Brenda *turned her attention* to *helping* him examine the effects of

drinking. *On the basis of that information, Charles decided* to
see a psychologist and eventually attended an alcohol counselling clinic.' (p. 21, emphasis added)

In this example, the patient Charles is introduced as an alcoholic of
long-standing who has been diagnosed with tuberculosis. He has
been placed on a therapeutic regime of medication to treat the
tuberculosis and Brenda, the community health nurse, is engaged in
a form of 'health promotion' which involves her actively monitor-
ing Charles' adherence to the medical regime.

In the example provided by Field, Charles is represented as
having made a choice not to take his medication. Field then goes on
to attribute all sorts of calculations made by Charles and Brenda
regarding this state of affairs. Charles, it is said, 'knows' that
drinking while taking medications for his tuberculosis is 'contra-
indicated'. Field's presentation of this encounter suggests that
Charles has no intention of ceasing his intake of alcohol. Field
describes him as having 'consciously decided' not to take the pills.

In relation to this portrayal of the patient, Brenda is represented
in the text as acknowledging his right to make such decisions. It
seems important (to Field) to suggest that Brenda does not press the
issue of the medication regime 'because' Charles has made a conscious decision. Instead, Brenda is said to turn her attention to
'helping' Charles 'examine the effects of his drinking'. Then, 'on the
basis of that information,' it is said that Charles 'decides' to seek
treatment for his drinking.

Read in this excruciatingly detailed way, this example seems
ready to explode with meanings. Yet in its original form, it is
'merely' a description of what was apparently observed by the field
researcher. There is no question that the nurse is doing health
promotion properly: it is a very settled example of practice. But
look again at what is said to have been observed: people making
'choices'; people 'turning' their attention elsewhere (from what?);
people making 'decisions' on the basis of information related to the
'effects' (social? physiological? moral?) of alcohol.

Clifford Geertz has reflected upon the impact that Wittgenstein's
Philosophical Investigations had on those (and he includes himself)
who believed 'that the answers to our most general questions –
why? how? what? whither? – to the degree they have answers, are

to be found in the fine detail of lived life' (Geertz, 2000: xi). He goes on to credit Wittgenstein as having launched an

'attack upon the idea of a private language, … [this attack] brought thought out of its grotto in the head into the public square where one could look at it.' (Geertz, 2000: xii)

Field's description of nursing practice is designed to leave thought locked up in that grotto of the mind. In her brief passage that seeks to give descriptive power to nursing practices of health promotion she leaves us in complete darkness as to the why, the how, the what and the whither of these intricate practices. Such opacity does nothing to help practising nurses make decisions about the directions they wish to follow in the interests of providing high-quality patient care. Instead, the description covers up the nurse's practices of powerful persuasion and her responses to the patient's practices of resistance to that persuasion.

I want to be clear here: I do not take Field's description as a 'poor' reporting of her research. Instead, it, like the practices of nurses I am interested in, must be read as an accomplishment of the work of nurses as power-neutral and the acquiescence of patients as something a 'good' nurse should be able to fully anticipate. The assumptions enabling this descriptive accomplishment stands in such opposition to the everyday world of contemporary nursing practice that it must be thoroughly challenged. Alternative practices for interpreting the materials collected while in the field can be imagined.

First, in order to spell out the challenge I wish to advance in relation to the form of fieldwork widely perpetuated within the nursing literature, I would like to focus on the very rational progression that is depicted through Field's choice of words. Field presents the practice event as a linear matter. It is as though Brenda was using one of the assessment 'guides' for her practice. The reader is required to imagine the context of the encounter. It seems that Brenda and Charles have met in some place where Brenda's legitimacy as a health care provider means that Charles is required, for a time at least, to share some aspects of his life and the choices he makes in living that life with Brenda. Within such an encounter, then, it seems that Brenda has discovered some 'problems' in need of her intervention: Charles has a 'drinking problem' and, tied up with this, he is making 'bad' decisions about medications prescribed for him by his physician.

In this example, Field proposes some significant, and I would argue, historically innovative positions for the nurse and for the 'client'. In terms of health promotion, what Field is 'advertising' here is what nurses might earlier have thought of as the 'correct move' for a health professional to take: that is, directing the patient to act in appropriate ways (e.g. 'Charles, you know that drinking is bad for your health. You should stop drinking and take your medication.'), should now be handled quite differently. Instead of telling patients what to do, Field suggests nurses should accept the 'consciously made' decisions of their patients. But Field does not leave the nurse without any interventions. The nurse is now advised by Field to 'turn her attention' elsewhere, perhaps to the underlying 'source' of the problem: the drinking. Field condenses what can only be imagined as quite a contentious and difficult conversation between Brenda and Charles about his alcoholism. But was it a conversation about Charles's alcoholism, or merely an abstract conversation about 'the effects of drinking' (Field, 1989: 21)? When Field claims that 'on the basis of this information' Charles makes a decision to seek alcohol counselling treatment, she glosses over the most significant part of this inter-action. Such glossing is, in my view, emblematic of nursing's long aversion to address the powerful effects of its practice. But it also signals that the analytic tools employed by Field to study and represent the practice of nurses are capable of treating such inter-ventions as entirely unproblematic.

It is worth noting that this summary of Field's much larger ethnographic study was published in a widely circulated 'trade' journal for nurses in Canada, *The Canadian Nurse*. It is the monthly publication of the Canadian Nurses Association, a national professional nursing organization. So, on the surface, the appearance of this article within that journal might be read as an endorsement of the value of research into nursing practice; it is also an endorsement of practice within a community setting. But the article conveys even more than this. Papers published in *The Canadian Nurse* are of a particular type. They are short, often opinion pieces, quite often 'edifying testimonials' (Nelson, 1997) about a nurse's work with a particular patient, perhaps seeing that patient through a difficult illness. And so, within this context, it is also possible to read the piece by Field as expressive of particular values regarding nursing practice: namely, that promoting health is a 'good' thing for nurses to be involved in and that no matter how difficult or intransigent the 'problems' facing a patient, a good nurse can help a patient see the right path to follow. A very optimistic picture of nursing and of patient care is expressed.

The lack of theoretical attention to power and resistance within a practice discipline such as nursing becomes increasingly frustrating and problematic as one considers the issues of power inherent within such examples of health-promoting interventions. Brenda, the nurse, is presented as someone assured of the appropriateness of her actions. There is no space in Field's account for uncertainty. Charles, the patient, is presented as someone needing only to be shown the logic of healthy action. Once clarified, he sets off on the 'right' path. The legitimacy of the health message and the docility of the response are remarkable – yet no space for remark is allowed within the text. Such treatment of nurse–patient encounters within the realm of health promotion, I argue, seriously underdetermines the agonistic (Lyotard, 1984) character of social relations. Under what conditions of practice can we understand such certainty and docility? Field's readings of practice arise out of and reinforce a view that practice is rational and linear. It denies the dynamic characteristics of health promotion as a highly contested field of practice and of health as a contested identity. Indeed, I would argue that the dynamism of practice has been stripped away in this account. Resolution of this issue of dynamism in reports of practice is not, however, simply a matter of addition. I am not suggesting that movement can somehow now be added back in and the issue will be resolved. The displacement of movement out of theoretical statements about nursing is an effect of the use of specific textual devices. The result, as the excerpt from Field's study exemplifies, is a conceptualization of practice as static. From this conceptual space, nurse theorists have been able to position themselves and their theoretical statements as 'necessary' for nurses to take up in order to situate themselves as rational practitioners equipped with rational tools that can be said to improve the status of (static) patients.

Setting practice in motion

The aim of my work over the past decade has been to develop a strong critique of the sort of research writing practices illustrated above. I am interested in seeking ways of tracing the effects of 'static views of social order that do not take account of the processes, ambiguities and differences involved in trying to think about the social ordering that we have come to call modernity' (Hetherington, 1997: vii). Alternative means for representing practice offer conceptualizations of humans as much less settled in their identities, much less sure of their actions and what they will lead to, struggling to be recognized. An example of such an alternative, and much more dynamic conceptualization is provided by the American anthropologist James Fernandez. Fernandez's view of human beings is that, rather than representing rational beings who progressively accumulate layers of knowledge, we are instead

> 'a very generalized animal with very little in specific adaptations to specific milieus wired into our brains. As a consequence we are required to invent ways of being – from rules and plans to worldviews and cosmologies – more or less appropriate to any of the diverse milieus in which we have installed ourselves. We endlessly argue over the appropriateness of those rules, plans, and worldviews. It may be a consequence of the self-conscious unrequitement implicit in the melancholy fact that, with great frequency, we fail to realize our rules and plans in the world . . . our reach so often exceeds our grasp.' (Fernandez, 1986: vii)

If we look back from this vantage point to Brenda's health-promoting action, we might see that her 'decision' to get around the situation presented to her by Charles was one in which she extended her reach in order to 'do promotion'. That such promotion of health was apparently achieved so easily stands in stark contrast to Fernandez's suggestion that 'our reach so often exceeds our grasp'. The question that remains unanswered in Field's description of practice is how did Charles come to decide to seek counselling? Was this extension into his life by Brenda accepted unproblematically by him? How did she accomplish this extension? I believe that Fernandez's representation of everyday action offers a way of exploring the dynamics of practice as nurses seek to express their professional identities as legitimate within the domain of health promotion. And I believe it offers analytic possibilities for examining the effects of that practice when it comes into relation with the contested terrain of health promotion.

Promoting health: a dynamic encounter

If I seek to approach materials collected in 'the field' and do that in such a way that I seek to maintain the dynamic character of those materials, I must approach them from a sufficiently robust theoretical location. For that, I turn again to Fernandez, who argues that, whether it is the business of interpreting research materials or of promoting health, I approach that work from a social location 'with very little in specific adaptations to specific milieus wired into [my] brain' (Fernandez, 1986: vii). Instead, I must 'invent' myself in ways that I take to be most appropriate, given my reading of the milieu I find myself in. To approach this sort of work in another way is to assume what Fernandez calls 'the dominant impulse in social science' which is

> 'that of *determining where people are rather than where they are going*. We want to put them in their place. We like to know their category. But however literal-mindedly men may classify themselves or be classified by category or by characteristic mood or temperament, they all fancy membership in other categories and undergo constant fluctuation in mood.' (Fernandez, 1986: 98, emphasis added)

Here, Fernandez keeps central that notion of 'argumentation' that, for him, cultivates dynamism in interpretation. Even when the most explicit rules are followed (by practitioners of all sorts), those whom we classify will argue that we have not quite got it 'right' and they will seek membership in other categories. It is this argumentation that I feel has most clearly been stripped away in Field's explication of Brenda's health-promoting practice.

An example from field notes taken within the context of another public health clinic in Canada will exemplify the effects of these positioning efforts. In this example we see a nurse, keen to promote the health of her identified subject, a baby brought to the clinic by his mother for routine immunization. We also see a mother keen to express herself as a competent and experienced parent.

This short excerpt is drawn from a 20-minute interaction between a public health nurse (Norma) and a client called Patti. Patti has brought her four-month old baby, Tom, and her 4-year old son, Pat, with her to the clinic. When they arrived at the clinic, Norma weighed and measured Tom and then invited Patti, who was carrying Tom and holding Pat's hand, into the office. They settled into their 'respective' seats (Norma near the desk in the swivel chair and Patti in the straight-backed chair by the door). Norma is about to 'interpret' the measurements she's taken of the baby to Patti.

> *Norma:* OK. This young man [Tom] ... is a big boy.
> *Patti:* Uh hmm.
> [Norma turns the graphic chart around so that Patti can see it. She illustrates with a pen where Tom's measurements show up on the graph.]
> *Norma:* Here's his, now I've put it in just that shade over the four months ...
> *Patti:* ... yeah ...
> *Norma:* ... and he's *ju-u-st* below the ninetieth percentile for length so he's moved up tremendously 'cause he was just above average ...
> *Patti:* ... yeah ...
> *Norma:* And his weight is just a bit below seventy-fifth so actually you can see that calorie growth has gone length-wise and he needs to fatten up a little. Eat a little bit more. Slow down his activity, whatever.
> [Patti laughs.]
> *Norma:* Yeah, sometimes that length will parallel off while the other ...
> *Patti:* Pat was always tall, he was always up in the ninety ...
> *Norma:* Yeah, well, he's certainly not underweight.
> [Norma glances over to where Pat is playing beside Patti's chair.]
> *Patti:* No, he's not suffering at all.

Norma: Head circumference maintaining up there around the ninetieth so ... he's [Tom] a good sized boy.

Perhaps the first thing that might be done here is to compare this extract from a baby clinic visit with that of Field's account of health-promoting nursing practice. If 'optimism' and 'progress' are characteristic of modernity, then these two examples, textualized quite differently, surely represent discourses of high modernism.

Upon entering the clinic office, the location of what the nurses took to be their 'real' work in the clinic, Norma quickly shifts into work mode and is actively, but in a taken-for-granted manner, seeking to tell Patti where the baby *is* rather than where he is *going*. That is, she interprets the measurements taken in the waiting room as indicating that the baby is growing disproportionately, that this is not ideal and that a health-promoting intervention could be designed to rectify this situation. We can see in this way that Norma's practice is guided by a rational, problem-solving model through which she can divide the baby in a particular way (as one who is growing disproportionately) and, through this device, position Patti to be susceptible to her health-promoting intervention. But this is where the rational model 'breaks down'. Instead of being positioned by Norma's manoeuvres, Patti resists being positioned: she treats Norma's suggestion as a joke. Norma's reach has exceeded her grasp – having extended herself this far, her identity as an expert is now in question. Fernandez (1986: 79) sees humour as a very particular mode of argumentation:

'It is in the nature of humour to make a sudden movement or set of movements in the face of our composure and settledness of situation ... We are frustrated because a customary domain of activity for which we are prepared ... suddenly gives evidence of elements belonging to another domain for which we are unprepared. In this shifting of domains our identities ... [are] brought into question. The joke depends upon the fact that we are never fully sure of our identity in any domain of life.'

Indeed, Norma's well-laid plan is upset; her 'settledness' as the health-promoting 'expert' in the clinic is upset; her predication of self within the encounter is completely disrupted.

And yet, miraculously, the situation does not dissolve. Rather, it is 'rescued' by Patti. While Patti rejects Norma's interpretation of the measurements as indicating something has gone wrong with her child's development, she has no intention of debunking the entire encounter.[2] She offers Norma an alternative explanation: 'Pat was always tall, he was up in the 90 . . .'. She uses Norma's own grounds to indicate that her children are 'all' like this. It's normal. And, fortunately she has the 'evidence' right at hand. Her older son has accompanied her to the clinic and, as they both agree, 'he's certainly not underweight', 'he's not suffering'. At this, Norma retreats. She legitimates her withdrawal by bringing into play the other measurement: the baby's head circumference. She ends the session – Tom's a good sized boy – he does not need fattening up or slowing down after all.

Extensions and overextensions

What is at stake in describing nursing practice as dynamic? First, and foremost: the nurse's power to define her own identity as central and constitutional of the nursing encounter. Second, the extent to which choices made by patients position nurses in ways that are just as potentially problematic as are the choices made by nurses in positioning patients. Each of these will be explored in turn.

While nurses' practices signal an expectation they hold that they have control over the constitution of a nursing encounter, the literature has been silent in investigating the implications of this expectation. Field studies of nursing practice that illustrate how *provisional* identity is – the identity of the nurse as well as of the patient – provide a context within which these constitutional matters could be raised up for detailed scrutiny and discussion. Such investigation, however, relies on an understanding that both parties (nurses and patients) are engaged in relations of commitment: 'in expressing ourselves, we must commit ourselves to movement or some other speculative image' (Fernandez, 1986: 96).

Fernandez's point underlines the value both for researchers and for practitioners in studies of practice as 'movement.' In any encounter, when the nurse expresses herself *as a nurse*, she commits to movement. Organizational demand may suggest that her options for movement are very narrow (e.g. numbers of referrals for alcohol counselling and immunization rates must meet particular targets). But practices of resistance to these sorts of organizational demands throw open the doors of possibility regarding how a nurse might express herself in any given circumstance. Required here is an understanding of the constitution of nursing as a co-creation (Northrup, 1995; Northrup & Cody, 1998).

In the description of practice that takes place between Norma and Patti, the power to define and the power to resist flow back and forth between the participants. Neither can be said, once and for all, to be 'the most powerful' actor. So, if nursing's problem with power is that 'having' it troubles them, they need not worry: they do not 'have' it once and for all. In practice, power is 'in play'. Nurses have resources they can draw on to accomplish a powerful position in relation to the patient (Norma uses her diagram of the baby's 'development' to offer suggestions to Patti on how to be a good parent), but patients have resources too (Patti can point to her successful parenting of her older child who was 'always tall' and in this way, similar to the baby).

Of interest in the example described in the immunization clinic is that Norma learns that the promotion of health is too narrow a practice domain for her to operate within. With Patti's help she is able to 'go on' (Giddens, 1984) in the encounter and, having broadened her domain of practice to allow Patti some expertise as well, she translates her care of the child's body into the language of health promotion. In doing so, she pulls back somewhat from the radical separation of health-promoting talk as practice and turns to consider a more grounded access to practice: the body of the patient.

Field studies offer an effective research methodology that can conceptualize nursing as an active and knowledgeable social accomplishment. It permits an illustration of how organizational imperatives come to organize the reporting of nursing care in such ways that the radical separation between what nurses take to be their work and the actual work they are accomplishing are created. It also offers a space in which nurses can examine how they organize their own practice, how they place innovations into that practice, and offers a moment of critique to ask the question, 'who am I when I am nursing?'

Notes

1. I acknowledge and express gratitude for the many long conversations I have had with my colleague Deborah Northrup on the extensiveness of the effects of such separating language.
2. I am grateful for long and interesting conversations with Rolland Munro in which I was alerted to such evidence of 'rescue'.

References

AARN (1987) *A Proposal for Integrating Health and Wellness into Nursing Practice*. Edmonton, AB: Alberta Association of Registered Nurses.

Anderson, B., Hannah, K., Besner, J., Broad, E., Duggleby, W., Larsen, S., Mackenzie, W. & Reyes, L. (1994) Health information: nursing components. *Canadian Nurse* **90**(9): 33–5.

de la Cuesta, C. (1994) Marketing: a process in health visiting. *Journal of Advanced Nursing* **19**: 347–53.

Elias, N. & Kilminster, R. (1991) *The Symbol Theory*. Newbury Park, CA: Sage.

Fawcett, J. (1995) *Analysis and Evaluation of Conceptual Models of Nursing*, 3rd edn. Philadelphia, PA: F.A. Davis.

Fernandez, J.W. (1986) *Persuasions and Performances: The Play of Tropes in Culture*. Bloomington, IN: Indiana University Press.

Field, P.A. (1989) Brenda, Beth and Susan. *Canadian Nurse* **85**(5): 20–24.

Geertz, C. (2000) *Available Light: Anthropological Reflections on Philosophical Topics*. Princeton, NJ: Princeton University Press.

Giddens, A. (1984) *The Constitution of Society*. Cambridge: Polity Press.

Glaser, B.G. & Strauss, A. (1967) *Discovery of Grounded Theory: Strategies for Qualitative Research*. Chicago: Aldine.

Goffman, E. (1974) *Frame Analysis*. Boston, MA: Northeastern University Press.

Gottlieb, L. (1981) Nursing clients toward health: an analysis of nursing interventions. *Nursing Papers/Perspectives on Nursing* **13**(1): 24–31.

Hetherington, K. (1997) *The Badlands of Modernity: Heterotopia and Social Ordering*. London: Routledge.

Latimer, J. (1995) The nursing process re-examined: enrolment and translation. *Journal of Advanced Nursing* **22**: 213–20.

Liepert, B. (1999) Women's health and the practice of public health nursing in British Columbia. *Public Health Nursing* **16**: 280–89.

Lindsey, E. & Hartrick, G. (1996) Health-promoting nursing practice: the demise of the nursing process?, *Journal of Advanced Nursing* 23: 106–12.

Lyotard, J-F. (1984) *The Postmodern Condition: A report on Knowledge* (G. Bennington & B. Massumi, trans), Vol. 10. Manchester: Manchester University Press.

Meleis, A.I. (1990) Being and becoming healthy: the core of nursing knowledge. *Nursing Science Quarterly* 3(3): 107–14.

Nelson, S. (1997) Reading nursing history. *Nursing Inquiry* 4: 229–36.

Northrup, D.T. (1995) Exploring the experience of time passing for persons with HIV disease: Parse's theory guided research. PhD dissertation, University of Texas at Austin, Austin.

Northrup, D.T. & Cody, W.K. (1998) Evaluation of the human becoming theory in practice in an acute care psychiatric setting. *Nursing Science Quarterly* 11(1): 23–30.

O'Brien-Pallas, L. & Baumann, A. (2000) Toward evidence-based policy decision: a case study of nursing health human resources in Ontario. *Nursing Inquiry* 7(4): 248–57.

Pender, N. (1987) *Health Promotion in Nursing Practice*, 2nd edn. East Norwalk, CT: Appleton & Lange.

Petersen, A. & Lupton, D. (1996) *The New Public Health: Health and Self in the Age of Risk*. St Leonards, NSW: Allen & Unwin.

Purkis, M.E. (2001) Governing the health of populations: the child, the clinic and the 'conversation'. In V. Hayes & L. Young (eds) *Transforming Health Promotion Practice: Concepts, Issues and Applications*. Los Angeles, CA: F.A. Davis, pp. 190–206.

Roy, C. (1984) *Introduction to Nursing: An Adaptation Model*, 2nd edn. Englewood Cliffs, NJ: Prentice Hall.

Stewart, M.J. (1995) *Community Nursing. Promoting Canadians' Health*. Toronto, ON: W.B. Saunders.

Strathern, M. (1991) *Partial Connections*, 3rd edn (Association for Social Anthropology in Oceania special publication). Savage, MD: Rowman & Littlefield.

Strauss, A. & Corbin, J. (1997) *Grounded Theory in Practice*. Thousand Oaks, CA: Sage.

Vollstedt, I. (1999) Social distancing between nurse and patient. PhD dissertation, University of Edinburgh, Scotland.

PART II

Selves

Practising nurses are interactionists: when they work with patients they are using many different aspects of themselves to know what patients need. So too are qualitative researchers. We can think of some of this knowing as embodied and as reflexive. The two chapters in this part explore and develop the epistemological underpinnings of participant observation as a research approach that engages the researcher as both subject and research instrument.

The problem of other minds has long vexed philosophers and social scientists alike. For nurses there is an assumption, sometimes explicit, but more often than not implicit, that there is a possibility that they need to know or understand from another's point of view: that they can, and that they should, as Jan Savage puts it, stand in the shoes of the other. Methods for developing nurses' skills and approach are advanced by nurse theorists and educationalists, which supposedly enable nurses to enter the world occupied by another in order to have some idea about how it is experienced by them. We have already seen in the chapter by Purkis, that there are many constraints on nurses simply entering the world of their patients and changing it. But what we have also seen is that knowing engages nurses as subjects in relations with their patients as subjects.

Field researchers also figure the relation between the researcher and the researched as a source of knowledge and understanding. The researcher is to enter the lives of a group of others in order to understand them, and some of this understanding depends upon the researchers seeing, feeling or thinking the world from the point of view of the researched in order to understand what they mean and why they do what they do.

The chapters in Part II draw out how, through participation in the world of the researched, researchers can understand and generate knowledge about their research subjects. However, each author explicates how this process is not straightforward. The chapters discuss how the act of participation in order to understand from the perspectives of others, and in order to know what it is that they know, is deeply problematic. While both authors argue for participation and immersion in the lived world of the other, as method, both authors illuminate how access and participation are mediated in complex ways which require reflection and the development of analytic and practical strategies.

CHAPTER 4

Participative observation: using the subject body to understand nursing practice

Jan Savage

In this chapter, I explore the idea that by standing in the place of research informants, by adopting their bodily practices, the researcher can gain access to their informants' experiential world. I call this approach 'participative observation'.

Nursing rests on many different ways of knowing, much of it derived directly from clinical practice, and a great deal of it concerned with the body and embodiment (Benner, 1984; Benner & Wrubel, 1989; Lawler, 1991; Parker, 1995). Nurses' intimacy with the patient's body, for example, is thought to provide special access to the patient's subjective world and embodied existence (Lawler, 1991). Rather differently, nurses' understanding of care, as in the philosophy of 'new nursing'[1] for instance, can inform and be expressed through the comportment and gestures that come to characterise their practice (Savage, 1999). However, such experiential knowledge or embodied intelligence has been widely dismissed within and beyond nursing. This is largely because these forms of knowing are not amenable to traditional forms of supposedly objective investigation that privilege what can be seen, measured and verbalised (Lawler, 1997b, c). As Lawler (1991) has put it, the lived body has been a casualty of nursing's ambition to be consistent with other disciplines through the scientising of practice.

There are compelling reasons why we need to find ways of articulating the experiential forms of knowledge that nurses (and some other health care practitioners) acquire. As Benner and Wrubel (1989) have pointed out, embodied intelligence is important for skilled nursing practice. Making clinical judgements, for example, may depend in part on the use of taken-for-granted bodily skills, such as ways of using a probe or attention to smell (Benner & Wrubel, 1989), that are employed without deliberate thought or reflection. Highlighting the role of such embodied intelligence in clinical decision making seems particularly relevant in the context of widespread concern in health care systems, such as the UK's National Health Service (NHS), that treatment and health care more generally should become 'evidence-based'. The establishment of the UK's new National Institute for Clinical Excellence (NICE), for example, represents a major shift in the conceptualisation and delivery of health care. Its main concerns are to ensure excellence in health care by making sure that all clinical decisions are based on 'sound evidence', that unexplained variations in treatment are eliminated, and that all treatments are cost effective (Loughlin, 2000).

While no one would wish to argue for a less than excellent service, initiatives like NICE raise potential problems for nursing. First, 'sound evidence' is assumed to be best provided by quantitative research, in particular the randomised controlled trial (RCT), on the basis that it provides precise, unambiguous and objective data. However, not everyone would agree that RCTs provide reliable results even within the terms of scientific or experimental inquiry (Charlton, 2000),[2] or that all aspects of treatment or patient care are amenable to scientific investigation.[3]

Second, the push for evidence-based practice has been seen to be driven less by the goal of excellence, and more by the political aim of enabling health service managers to control the judgement and decision-making processes of clinicians (Charlton, 2000). On this basis it seems important to challenge the concept of 'evidence', and to find ways of articulating the non-measurable elements of quality health care, such as embodied intelligence, and the ambiguities of practice, if nurses are to resist attempts to undermine their professional autonomy. Because of the complex nature of nursing, finding more appropriate ways of exploring nursing knowledge demands a careful balance of new and existing methodologies, and awareness of the limitations of those methodologies borrowed from other disciplines (Lawler, 1997c: 49). With this caution in mind, this chapter explores the potential offered to nurses by 'participative observation'.

Participative observation is the explicit attempt to learn

through the body and make bodily participation and use of the senses central to the collection and interpretation of data. As a form of participant observation, it draws on a pre-existing body of knowledge generated by social scientists, particularly anthropologists and sociologists. At the same time, in its focus on embodied intelligence, and its assumptions about what can be learnt from and through the body, participative observation shares some of the issues and assumptions that inform nursing (Savage, 2000).

Both endeavours, nursing and participative observation, raise important questions about the distinction between subjective and objective experience, and about the distinction between self and other. The project of nursing, for example, is seen to require 'a sufficient projection of self into the private world of the other [the patient], to be able (at least partially) to understand effectively what the experience means for them' (Brykcznska, 1992: 6) (emphasis in original). Similarly, Benner (1984: 4) argues that the act of caring 'places the person [nurse] in the situation [of the patient] in such a way that certain aspects show up as relevant' (emphasis added). Not so differently, in the more participative forms of participant observation, Jorgensen (1989: 63) suggests that researchers can 'become the phenomenon' under study and experience it existentially. As Jackson (1989: 9) has put it:

> 'We must come to [knowledge] through participation as well as observation and not dismiss lived experience ... as "interference" or "noise" to be filtered out in the process of creating an objective report for our profession.'

Thus, amongst practitioners of both nursing and participant observation there are those who suggest that interacting individuals can stand in each other's shoes and experience the world from the other's perspective. This 'standing in' for, or as, the other, however, is not purely a figure of speech, but refers to the capacity of the embodied self to understand those regarded as other through physical involvement in their world. After a brief discussion of the role of the participative body in nursing and in research, the chapter considers some of the epistemological issues that 'participative observation' raises, before discussing the use of this approach through an example from research.

Bodies in nursing

According to Lawler (1997c), nursing knowledge has been devalued because of what she refers to as 'the problem of the body' – the way in which the body and its functions, despite being central to our existence, remains obscure. Lawler suggests that this is due in part to the way in which an emphasis on empiricism has led to a theoretical fragmentation of corporeal and embodied existence:

> 'The "problem of the body" means ... that although a social and human body is integral to our existence, no discipline has yet overtly, explicitly and theoretically accommodated it, except in pieces. The body has been subjected to reduction and so too has our knowledge and experience of the body in social life.' (Lawler, 1991: 2)

Yet, although the body or embodied existence has, until very recently, been little more than implicit in orthodox nursing discourse, in many forms of nursing practice the body is known in a way that integrates mind and body, and which emphasises the embodied nature of everyday life (Lawler, 1991). New scholarship in nursing is beginning to articulate the presence of the body in nursing.[4] However, so far, this has tended to focus on the kind of knowledge that nurses can develop with regard to their patients' experience of an ailing or compromised body. Lawler (1991: 29), for instance, has described what she refers to as 'somology' in terms of nurses' understanding of the patient's body as simultaneously an object, a means of experience, a manner of presence among other people, and a part of one's personal identity. There is also growing interest in the way that the body provides a focus in the nurse–patient relationship and 'what takes place between the nurse and the patient as people who are often situated as captives together' (Lawler, 1997a: 33). Rudge's (1996) work on the abject experience of patients with burns and of the nurses who work with them, provides an important example of this. We also have moving insights into what it means to receive bodily care, and the significance of the nurse's own body in this, from people who have been patients.

For example, Albie Sachs's (1990) account of his recovery after becoming the target of a car bomb describes the way that healing meant not only coming to terms with severe injuries, but also facing the fact that these were deliberately inflicted. In this he felt that the physical involvement of nurses, and others such as physiotherapists, indicated their commitment to his healing. It was not just through words, but through their bodily actions and presence, that nurses expressed their support in what Sachs describes as a physical giving of self in a professional setting. Yet, so far, this physical giving of self has rarely been considered in any detail from the nurse's per-spective: we have little knowledge of nurses' lived experience of their own bodies as constituted through practice.

Perhaps one reason for this silence about the nurse's body is the methodological difficulties raised by attempts to research the body and embodiment, and to articulate lived experience. However, these difficulties have received consideration by a number of researchers beyond nursing who, as suggested earlier, have begun to explore the potential of participant observation to use the embodied self of the researcher as a means of accessing the experiential world of others.

Bodies in participant observation

It is difficult to talk about any form of participant observation without first some mention of ethnography, particularly as the terms are often used interchangeably. There are those who suggest, for example, that besides ethnography, other terms ... also cover the same procedure – fieldwork, qualitative sociology, participant observation, and what Geertz called 'thick description'. All aim at a method that is imbued with many interpretive strands and layers, committed in some measure to reconstructing the actor's own world-view (Rock, 2001: 30). In this chapter, however, I start from the premise that ethnography is not a procedure or method, but is both a research product (a text) and a methodology.

As a methodology, or a theoretically informed approach (Ellen, 1984), ethnography has been the subject of lengthy debate. For some such as Lincoln and Denzin (1994), its traditional form has been influenced by the principles of realism and assumptions about the privileged nature of the ethnographer's gaze. In contrast, contemporary forms of ethnography recognise the possibility of multiple 'realities', and the complexity of the relationships that exist between the researcher and the researched. Others doubt that the history of ethnography has been marked by discrete phases of positivism and modernism but that instead 'there has been a repeated dialectic between what might be thought of as a dominant orthodoxy, and other, centrifugal forces that have promoted difference and diversity' (Atkinson *et al.*, 2001:3).

Strangely, participant observation, often assumed to be a cornerstone of ethnography, has remained of marginal interest in this debate in as much as the epistemological assumptions that underpin its use are rarely explored. It has been suggested, for example, that participant observers take on a dual role, both as participants who 'feel, hear and see a little of social life as one's subjects do', and observers who remain 'ultimately distinct and objectifying' (Rock, 2001: 32). But this understanding of participant observation assumes that objective observation is possible, and that the nature of the relationship between the participant observer and research informants is unproblematic (Tonkin, 1984). Moreover, it is often accompanied by an assumption, dating back to the Ancient Greeks, that what is 'objectively' observed will have greater epistemological value than data generated by other senses (Grosz, 1994).

Championed for its detachment by rationalists and empiricists such as Descartes and Locke, sight has been the principal sense employed in science, and influential in the development of a mode of thought that emphasises detachment (Classen, 1993). As Jackson (1989) has argued, an 'ocularcentric' way of knowing implies an assumption of distance between the knower and the known that allows one to be an impartial observer and the other to be subject to the observer's gaze. The inherent power of the observer has become recognised by philosophers and social scientists such as Sartre (1984) in his exposé of the sadomasochism intrinsic to 'the look', and Foucault (1973: 89), who demonstrates the sovereignty of the gaze in science, suggesting that it is 'the eye that knows and decides, the eye that governs'.

The privileging of sight, or what Jay (1999) has called the 'hegemony of vision', may therefore have important implications for health care practitioners and researchers. For example, the powerful nature of the gaze raises questions about observation as an appropriate approach for health care issues in the current ethos that promotes partnership between researchers and research participants (see, for instance, Department of Health, 2000). However, not everyone would agree that it is advisable, or even possible, for the researcher to remain distant or detached. Davies (1999), for example, points out that if scientists such as astronomers question the interaction between themselves and the focus of their observation, distant stellar events, the problematic nature of detachment must be especially relevant to social researchers who work with conscious and self-aware beings.

In addition, it cannot be assumed that there is a clear boundary between the external and internal worlds of the researcher: as Herdt (1990: 36) has put it, it is not always possible to distinguish 'between events in the world [and] those in the head of the ethnographer'. Yet the very idea of an internal world as events in the head of the ethnographer suggests a further distinction, an assumption of a cerebral form of cognition that neglects the role of the body in knowing.

Following the work of philosophers such as Merleau-Ponty (1962), it is now more commonly recognised that we inhabit the world through our embodied interactions, and that it is through our bodies that we are able to understand this world. As Leder (1992: 25) has put it, we cannot understand those things external and separate to us without reference to bodily powers through which we engage them – our senses, motility, language, desires. The lived body is not just one thing in the world but a way in which the world comes to be.

Despite increased awareness of the importance of the lived body in understanding the world, however, there is still little discussion of the theoretical premises that will inform the way that embodiment is studied, or the nature of the knowledge it affords us. For example, in participant observation that aims to utilise all the senses in data collection (see Stoller, 1997, for instance), the underlying assumption appears to be that the researcher can acquire understandings of cultural practices and local knowledge[5] that are generally not verbalised by becoming the subject of study through physically enacting the life of the 'other'. This suggestion appears similar, at least to some extent, to the idea of mimesis that has been posited as central to the process of knowing and the construction of identities (Taussig, 1993).

According to Taussig, the mimetic faculty is the capacity to imitate and become 'other'. More specifically, the imitation 'draw[s] on the character and power of the original to the point whereby the representation may even assume that character and power' (Taussig, 1993: xiii). It is probably true to say that this mimetic faculty is not employed in most forms of participant observation, but it is assumed to come into play with what I call 'participative observation' in order not simply to talk about the body but, as Farnell (2000: 413) has put it, to 'talk from the body'.

Participative observation

The difference between participative observation and participant observation can be illustrated using the following account by an anthropologist (Gregor, 1977: 28) in which he explains a shift in his fieldwork strategy to understand the lives of certain Brazilian Indians. Gregor (1977: 28) describes why he went from accompanying the village men on fishing and hunting expeditions to carrying out household surveys in the following terms:

> 'Every day I would come back from treks through the forest numb with fatigue, ill with hunger, and covered with ticks and biting insects. My own work was difficult to pursue, for there is no time to pester men at work with irrelevant questions about their mother's brother.'

Here it appears that understanding of the kinship domain was thought best attained by the collection of ostensibly 'objective' information by asking, for example, who lived where and with whom. It might be argued, however, that Gregor could have centralised his participative role, through which he came to know the everyday hardships shared by men in the search for food, to attain a more fundamental understanding of the organisation and meaning of relationships amongst villagers. Yet this approach assumes that 'the body is an important point of departure for any process of knowing' (Rudberg, 1997: 182). As such, it raises an important question of whether what is learnt by or through the body can be shared by others inhabiting different bodies. One way of considering this question is through the work of Bourdieu and his concept of 'habitus' in explaining the way that bodily practices become shared and meaningful within social groups.

Theoretical stance

According to Bourdieu (1990), the practices that we enact in everyday life, such as ways of standing, speaking, walking and thereby of feeling and thinking, embody the fundamental, structuring principles of the social groups to which we belong. The nature of these value-bearing, quasi-bodily dispositions (what Bourdieu calls 'habitus')[6] is clarified by Bourdieu's descriptions of the Kabyle people of Algeria, with whom he worked for some time as an anthropologist.

Amongst the Kabyle, according to Bourdieu, an opposition between male and female is associated with a similar polarisation of certain social values (for example, straight/bent; directness/reserve; firmness/flexibility) that are made flesh through posture and the movements or gestures of the body. Thus a Kabyle man 'is like the heather, he would rather break than bend' – he stands straight and looks directly in the face of the person he meets. In contrast, a Kabyle woman is expected to walk with a slight stoop, looking downward and averting her eyes from others:

> 'In short, the specifically feminine virtue, lah'ia, modesty, restraint, reserve, orients the whole female body downwards, towards the ground, the inside, the house, whereas male excellence, nif, is asserted in movements upwards, outwards, towards other men.' (Bourdieu, 1990: 70)

According to Bourdieu, the structuring principles of *lah'ia* and *nif* are translated into the practical actions of men and women, as demonstrated by the Kabyle division of labour. In harvesting olives, for example, men stand and knock down olives from the trees with a pole, while women stoop to gather the fallen olives from the ground.

Of particular relevance to this chapter is Bourdieu's assertion that the body does not acquire culturally specific dispositions by deliberate imitation – that would presuppose a conscious effort to reproduce gestures, posture, movement and so on.[7] Instead, the child or the social novice attains practical mastery through the reproduction of other people's actions, a form of learning that is transmitted or acquired without calculation, but in or through practice, without resort to speech. Thus 'what is "learnt by the body" is not something that one has, like knowledge that can be brandished, but something that one is' (Bourdieu, 1990: 73). Nor do these practices become habitual as the result of explicit rules: as Bourdieu (1990: 53) puts it, dispositions 'can be collectively orchestrated without being the product of the organising action of a conductor'. Instead, a group's structuring principles are 'made body by the hidden persuasion of an implicit pedagogy which can instil a whole cosmology, through injunctions as insignificant as "sit up straight" or "don't hold your knife in your left hand"' (Bourdieu, 1990: 69). Thus, the fundamental principles and values of a culture are inscribed in the seemingly insignificant details of bodily and verbal etiquette.

The kind of unspoken instruction that Bourdieu refers to is powerfully brought to light by the following account of how bodily dispositions and social values – in this case, about women and sexuality – are learnt. This is extracted from work published by a group of German women who explored the socialisation of the body through studying photographs of their childhood and the memories that these prompted (Haug *et al.*, 1987). One particular woman, in describing the memories rekindled by a photograph of herself with her brother and sister, suggests something of the way in which habitus is acquired.

'He and I are sitting "like two young louts", my mother says. My sister, quite proper, chaste, obedient, sits with her legs closed, carefully placed one beside the other. I still have a clear memory of the moment when the picture was taken – I was barely five years old – and the sense of triumphant defiance when, at the very last moment before the picture was taken, I could no longer be prevented from sitting with my legs spread-eagled, the image of this unseemly behaviour captured forever on film. Nowadays I realise that this feeling, this attitude of the body, of the legs, cannot so easily be expressed in the way I felt then, as proof of independence, as a refusal of obedience, as resistant to the way I had been brought up to behave. Whatever I say about my legs [now] – that they are spread-eagled, spread apart, not closed – has an aftertaste of something disreputable, something obscene, it is coloured with sexual overtones. If I want to avoid this I have to talk, not of legs, but of a whole person, whom I describe as loutish or boorish ... and yet I know very well that everything began with my legs.' (Haug *et al.*, 1987: 75)

Haug *et al.* (1987), in reflecting on this account, observe that the imperative for 'nice girls' to keep their knees together is presented as a matter of orderliness, with no explicit reference to the sexual connotations attached to women who sit with their legs apart. Yet, they suggest, even if a young girl had no precise understanding of her parents' words on how to sit, it is likely that she would sense from their tone and manner that they are referring to a matter of considerable significance. In this way, 'sexualisation is acquired without sexuality itself ever being mentioned' (Haug *et al.*, 1987: 77). This example of the way in which habitus is acquired fits neatly with Bourdieu's (1990: 69) suggestion that 'arms and legs are full of numb imperatives'. However, the reference to numb imperatives also hints at criticisms of Bourdieu's theory on habitus that are relevant to participative observation. These concern the nature and location of human agency.

In suggesting that the body is a mnemonic device on which socio-cultural imperatives have been written, Bourdieu's concept of habitus has been critiqued as in essence Cartesian in that it separates the body and its dispositions from the mind and from discourse. Thought is implied to be divorced from action by assuming action is unconscious if not linked with self-reflective, propositional thought (Farnell, 2000). Farnell clarifies this point through using the example of 'knowing' how to ride a bicycle. She suggests that most people cannot describe how to ride a bike, or articulate the laws of physics on which this action rests. In other words, 'knowing' something does not imply a corresponding ability to talk about what is known. According to Farnell, Bourdieu's mistake is to assume that lack of ability to talk about certain kinds of knowledge means a lack of consciousness. Moreover,

> 'The conception of habitus denies the possibility of thoughtful action because it limits the body to its Cartesian status, a mindless, unconscious repository and mechanistic operator of practical techniques.' (Farnell, 2000: 409)

However, it could be countered that the lived body can never be fully explicit. Leder (1990: 1), for example, notes the highly paradoxical nature of bodily presence:

> 'While in one sense the body is the most abiding and inescapable presence in our lives, it is also essentially characterised by its absence. That is, one's own body is rarely the thematic object of experience.'

He gives the example of how, when reading a book, the reader generally loses most awareness of their bodily state. This is despite the fact that the body is the medium by which the reader's world comes into being. This absence, Leder argues, is an intrinsic tendency of the body, although exaggerated within western cultural traditions. If this is the case, it would suggest that, rather than Bourdieu's concept of habitus being unable to explain thoughtful action, that the difficulty lies more within the lived body that Bourdieu has tried to describe, and what Leder has termed the body's principle of absence. This is not to deny the possibility of embodied consciousness, but to suggest that such consciousness is contexual and inconstant. We become aware of our bodies, for example, in ageing, illness or other changes in circumstance. According to Young (1990), being pregnant represents a prime example of being thrown into awareness of one's own body, while Frank (1991: 51) suggests that 'the body becomes most conscious of itself when it encounters resistance, which is to say, when it is in use, acting'.

This discussion of embodied consciousness is necessarily limited,[8] but hopefully has been sufficient to allow consideration of some of the issues raised by participative observation.

Participative observation and thoughtful action

There are a number of different ways in which the experience of the lived body has been drawn upon in research. The anthropologist

Judith Okely (1992: 16) notes how the writing of field notes sometimes acts as a trigger for 'bodily and hitherto subconscious memories' that constitute a form of knowledge. This knowledge, she suggests, cannot be written about at the time, only in retrospect, when it helps to 'make sense' of written accounts. The body can thus, as Bourdieu (1977: 94) suggests, be treated 'as a memory'.

In addition, Okely (1994) has found that participant observation in the physical labour of others, in her case activities such as potato picking or milking cows, has provided major breakthroughs in understanding. She suggests that, through participation, the field-worker begins to respond to the patterns and rhythms that exist in the field of study. Okely provides one example of this response from her work among Traveller Gypsies to show how she became aware of the way in which, over time, her stance had become attuned to that of the Travellers. Seeing a photograph of herself and a Traveller woman that was taken by a stranger, she notes how 'I have unknowingly imitated the Gypsy woman's defensive body posture. We are both standing with arms folded, looking away from the lens' (Okely, 1992: 17). In this stance, Okely finds herself living the tension between the Travellers and Gorgios or members of the dominant, settled population from whom they are keen to remain separate.

In contrast, some fieldworkers deliberately set out to use their own body as a means of access to the world of others. An example of this approach is provided by the work of Lærke (1998) who, in an ethnographic study of an English village, focused particularly on the world views of children. She was concerned to use an approach that recognised children as active social agents rather than passive recipients of a predetermined social world. She therefore decided as a researcher to 'destabalise' or compromise her position as an adult and engage directly with children by placing herself, as far as possible, in the same physical and social space as them. She moved into the world of being small through, for example, dressing in similar ways to the children, relating to teachers as children did, sitting on the floor or in small chairs at school, and asking adults for things she needed that were beyond the reach of children. As a consequence she found that '[her] body was re-arranged, re-inscribed with sensations, perspectives and movements which I associated with my childhood' (Lærke, 1998: 3–4).

Lærke is keen to point out that her presence with children did not simply elicit fixed memories of her childhood, unaltered by her life during the intervening years, which she could project onto the children in her study:

> 'The children were both other than and same as me; in the process of my fieldwork socialisation, this simultaneous otherness and sameness was expressed as a tension between my past and present.' (1998: 5)

However, using her personal history as a methodological tool allowed her to catch glimpses of what it was like to be a child in a way that direct questioning did not. This approach to fieldwork, using the embodied self[9] to study others, is also taken up by the protagonists of 'sensual anthropology' (Stoller, 1997) or 'radical empiricism' (Jackson, 1989).

Jackson, for example, argues that knowledge is often embedded in practices rather than speech, and that an empathic understanding of this practical knowledge can be gleaned by the participant observer through the imitation of the other's bodily actions. In this, Jackson draws on Bourdieu's concept of habitus and his suggestion that the process by which habitus is acquired is two-way. Not only are social dispositions inscribed on the body as postures and gestures, but the body acts as a storehouse of suspended thoughts or feelings that can be recovered by adopting the postures or gestures that embody these. According to Bourdieu, this is not a matter of the body remembering, but of its enacting the past. As an example of this approach, Jackson describes how, when he went to live with the Kuranko of Sierra Leone as an anthropologist, he assumed that lighting his own fire for cooking and boiling water had little relevance for his research. But through observing Kuranko women over time, he became aware of their very precise techniques for building and lighting fires. By adopting their actions, he realised that these techniques had not only an aesthetic quality, but also a practical basis in that they allowed the best use of scarce firewood, making cooking more efficient by enabling control of the fire's intensity. In other words, through imitating certain Kuranko practices, Jackson believed that he had acquired a degree of Kuranko non-verbalised, commonsense knowledge.

It was after reading Jackson's work that I became interested in applying this kind of participative observation to nursing practice, to try to gain access to non-verbalised knowledge that I assumed was implicit in nurses' bodily practices. The next section describes the process of using participative observation during the routine bedside handovers that formed part of a study of nurse–patient interaction, with a view to exploring some of the issues raised by this approach for nurse researchers.

Participative observation in a study of nurse–patient interaction

Ethnographic research was carried out on a 17-bedded ward where primary nursing was used to care for patients with chronic medical and surgical gastro-intestinal conditions. All patients were male, and all nurses (apart from one student nurse and one health care assistant) were female. The study aimed to understand the nature and implications of nurse–patient interaction in which 'closeness' was encouraged on the basis that it could help bring about radical changes in practice (Pearson, 1988). It had previously been believed that nurses often remained distant from their patients in an attempt to protect themselves from anxiety (Menzies, 1970). The study was therefore concerned to explore the meaning of 'closeness' and identify whether nurses on this ward were adequately supported if they developed 'close' relationships with patients (see Savage, 1995, 1997).

Attempts to use participative observation were limited because I had not practised as a nurse for some time and was not competent to attempt many aspects of the nurses' work. My participation was, therefore, confined to activities such as bathing patients, talking with patients, fetching and carrying, and generally trying to make myself useful. I also participated in activities such as weekly ward meetings, and the handover at the start of every new shift when nurses passed on information about patients to oncoming staff.

It emerged that, for many nurses on the research ward, 'closeness' meant an emotional connection, often brought about by an exchange of confidences (sometimes reciprocal) between nurse and patient. This emotional intimacy was facilitated by the physical closeness that nurses encouraged between themselves and their patients. Apart from the proximity inherent in nurses' care of the patient's body, nurses further destabilised the boundary between themselves and their patients by dismantling their own private space. The overriding aim was to spend as much time as possible with the patient. There was therefore no designated nursing office or nursing station, and teaching and the writing of care plans took place at the bedside.

In most interactions, nurses sat on or beside the patient's bed, and held the patient's hand in an almost routine manner. Patients appeared on the whole to be delighted by this proximity. At the same time, nurses working this 'closely' with patients expressed no need for support beyond what they already received from their patients and their peers on the ward. However, my experience of the handover suggests that, despite deconstructing the boundary between themselves and their patients as part of a strategy for the delivery of quality care (and perhaps a professional strategy – see Savage, 1997), nurses nonetheless found ways of marking their difference from patients. In other words, the boundary between nurses and patients was redrawn rather than wholly dismantled. This was most evident during the nursing handover which, like other aspects of practice, took place at the patient's bedside.

The nurses on the ward worked in three different teams, each with their own patients to ensure the maximum continuity of care. At the handover, the nurses who worked with a particular patient would settle themselves around him, with the emphasis on 'getting down to the patient's level'. Nurses therefore either sat on the bed or squatted or kneeled on the floor nearby. Moreover, looking at the ward overall, as each team of nurses rose from one bedside and sank down again at another, the handover became a kind of Mexican wave[10] that rippled around the ward in a scene reminiscent of Bourdieu's statement about dispositions being collectively orchestrated without the direction of a conductor. Apart from demonstrating the close nature of their relationships with patients, this 'wave' or collective undulation also drew attention to the suppleness or flexibility of the nurses. Besides emphasising their youth, it highlighted their good health in what was otherwise a space concerned with sickness. Thus, while nurses arguably demolished a boundary between themselves and their patients in terms of physical and emotional space to claim a closeness with patients that was not available to other professional groups, they nonetheless demonstrated their difference through emphasising their physical and social flexibility.

Flexibility, as a principle informing practice, presented subtle advantages for nurses with regard to patient care and professional strategy. For example, nurses on the ward prided themselves on their responsiveness and adaptability to patients' needs, while their medical colleagues, in contrast, were considered as formal or stiff in their dealings with patients, and unbending in their adherence to regimes and protocols (Savage, 1999). In terms of my participation in the handover, this was instructive in a way I had not anticipated.

Early on in fieldwork, rather than giving me access to the embodied world of the ward's nurses, my participation in the handover served to inform me of the differences between us, particularly that I was considerably older and less flexible (both physically and socially), than my colleagues. Unlike other nurses who moved gracefully from one position to another, I staggered from kneeling to standing. I felt stiff and awkward, particularly to begin with, when I felt that my lack of up-to-date knowledge (a lack that was inscribed on my body and expressed in my awkwardness) meant that I was not really a nurse. Significantly, I became more flexible and less clumsy with time, and came to remember something of my earlier lived experience as a nurse, when nursing competence was embodied in surer and more fluid movement. These glimpses of my earlier self, however, were relived in the context of a different, older body, with additional meanings and values inscribed upon it.

While participation in, and conscious imitation of, nurses' bodily practices in the handover largely served to emphasise my difference from nurses participating in the research, I also found that I adopted other practices apparently without thinking. For example, as mentioned earlier, nurses seemed to touch patients in an almost routine manner. In addition to instrumental uses of touch (for example in dressing a wound), or the use of touch to comfort an anxious or distressed patient, nurses would touch patients without any obvious professional reason except by way of greeting or establishing and maintaining 'closeness'. Initially I found this use of touch a little disturbing. If not intrusive, it seemed artificial or mawkish. However, over the months that I spent on the ward, although it was not something that I consciously set out to do, I found that I similarly used touch in this way with many patients, and felt entirely comfortable doing so. It was not that I used touch unconsciously – I was aware of when I was using it or when it seemed inappropriate – rather, I had not 'told myself' to use touch in this way, nor could I explain why it became appropriate.

Discussion

This chapter has been concerned with finding ways of accessing the embodied intelligence of nurses and has focused on what I have called 'participative observation' as a means of doing this. The literature in this field has suggested both that the body acts as a memory, or that knowledge can be reclaimed from the body on reflection, and that understanding the embodied knowledge of others can be facilitated by adopting their bodily practices or dis-positions. Jackson's (1989) radical empiricism, for example, can be understood as a form of participative observation in which the researcher sets out to consciously mimic the bodily dispositions of informants in order to gain access to knowledge that is not gener-ally brought to an explicit level of discussion.

Experience of using participative observation suggests an epis-temological problem with this approach in that such participation is flawed by the impossibility of deliberately shrugging off our per-sonal histories as researchers or subjects in our own right. It assumes that the embodied ways in which we carry and reconstruct our pasts can be stripped away to leave an essential experience of the body that exists independently of cultural, political or other meanings. As Farnell (1994: 937) has put it: 'to assume ... that the sheer fact of embodiment allows one to inhabit the world of the Other, is to reduce cultural body to biological organism'. As the example from the research on closeness suggests, even when mimicking the actions or movements of others, the researcher's body is not a *tabula rasa* on which the experiences of others can be inscribed, unmodified by those of the researcher.

In my attempts to use a participative approach to the study of a practice-based occupation such as nursing, my prior experience as a nurse meant that, to some extent, I came across similar issues to those raised by Lærke (1998): I was working with a group who in some ways were the same as me, and in some ways other. Just as Laerke had her own memories of being a child to draw from, so I had memories of nursing; yet just as her memories were inseparable from her status now as an adult, so my experience of nursing was re-embodied in a different, older person. In some ways, deliberately mimicking the practices of nurses on the ward served to highlight some of the differences between us, rather than allow me access to the nurses' subjective worlds. Yet, becoming aware of what constituted otherness in this context helped me to make aspects of these nurses' practice more explicit.

There have been other findings from the employment of participative observation indicating sufficient resonance between this approach, the practice of nursing, and Bourdieu's concept of habitus to justify further inquiry. For example, as a participative observer, I began to assume some of the bodily dispositions of nurses on the ward in a way that suggests I acquired some aspects of the nurses' habitus. This was clearest in the way that I unintentionally adopted what was, for me, a new way of using touch without meaning to do so – if anything, I originally intended to avoid using touch as other nurses did on the ward. However, although this departure from previous practice was not premeditated, it was not an unconscious development. I was aware that my use of touch was being shaped by what felt appropriate as an embodied subject, and influenced in part by what I knew of patients' expectations as well as broader (for example, professional) judgements about appropriateness.

This phenomenon of 'thoughtful action' is interesting in the context of critiques of Bourdieu's work arguing that the concept of habitus implicitly separates thought from action. It is also reminiscent of depictions of nursing practice elsewhere, and the way that practice can be understood as the outcome of a dialectical relationship between action and 'knowing how' (Jones, 1997). Aspects of nursing knowledge have been seen to be held bodily as a habit or skill, and reliant on bodily senses: as Benner has put it, nurses' knowledge accumulated through experience is expressed as skilful, ethical 'comportment' (Benner, 1991). From this it would appear that, just as Bourdieu argues that the body does not acquire special dispositions through deliberate imitation but through practice, the participative observer is unlikely to gain access to their informants' experiential world by imitating their bodily practices. But, through encouraging experience in the field, and promoting attention to the researcher's experiential world (such as whether or how he or she develops new 'dispositions', or some degree of skilled, ethical comportment), participative observation may hold the potential for new understandings of the embodied intelligence of nurses.

Acknowledgements

I would like to thank Joanna Latimer for her support and insightful comments during the development of this chapter. In addition, I remain grateful to the nurses in the study referred to here, for help and food for thought.

Notes

1. This can briefly be characterised as a patient-centred form of nursing that is both instrumental and emotionally expressive, put into effect through patterns of care such as primary nursing (Pearson, 1988). New nursing has also been seen to be compatible with the political agenda of nurses wishing to free nursing from the shadow of medicine, as well as that of managers hoping to clarify the responsibility of new members of staff (Bowers, 1989).
2. Charlton (2000), for example, argues that RCTs are conducted on unrepresentative populations of heterogeneous subjects.
3. The term 'scientific' is open to a number of different interpretations. In arguing for a greater role for the senses in the collection of ethnographic data, for example, Stoller (1989: 9) suggests: 'that considering the senses of taste, smell, and hearing as much as privileged sight will not only make ethnography more vivid and more accessible, but will render our accounts of others more faithful to the realities of the field – accounts that will then be more, rather than less, scientific'.
4. See, for example, contributions to Lawler, 1997a.
5. By this I mean the kind of knowledge constituted by practice, linked to specific locations and circumstances, and often more about 'knowing how' than 'knowing what' (Hobart, 1993).

6. Or, as Jenkins (1992: 74) explains, 'a habitual or typical condition, state or appearance, particularly of the body'.

7. Here Bourdieu is talking about something quite different to Taussig's view of mimesis. Taussig suggests the mimetic faculty to be 'the compulsion to become the Other' (1993: xviii), and implies that mimesis is more consciously sought.

8. For more detail, see Frank, 1991.

9. Or an embodied self, given the unstable nature of selfhood (Battaglia, 1995).

10. The Mexican wave gains its name from the practice of football match spectators, who stand and then sit in apparently synchronised sequence, to give the impression of a wave undulating around the stadium, a practice that I believe first came to general attention through television coverage of the Mexican World Cup Final.

References

Atkinson, P., Coffey, A., Delamont, S., Lofland, J. & Lofland, L. (eds) (2001) Editorial introduction. In *Handbook of Ethnography*. London: Sage, pp. 1–10.

Battaglia, D. (1995) Problematising the self: a thematic introduction. In D. Battaglia (ed.) *Rhetorics of Self-Making*. Berkeley, CA: University of California Press.

Benner, P. (1984) *From Novice to Expert: Excellence and Power in Clinical Nursing Practice*. Menlo Park, CA: Addison-Wesley.

Benner, P. (1991) The role of experience, narrative, and community in skilled, ethical comportment. *Advances in Nursing Science* 14(2): 1–21.

Benner, P. & Wrubel, J. (1989) *The Primacy of Caring: Stress and Coping in Health and Illness*. Menlo Park, CA: Addison-Wesley.

Bourdieu, P. (1977) *Outline of a Theory of Practice*. Cambridge: Cambridge University Press.

Bourdieu, P. (1990) Belief and the body. In *The Logic of Practice*. Oxford: Polity Press, pp. 66–79.

Bowers, L. (1989) The significance of primary nursing. *Journal of Advanced Nursing* 27: 730–36.

Brykczynska, G. (1992) Caring – a dying art? In M. Jolley & G. Brykczynska (eds) *Nursing Care: The Challenge to Change*. London: Edward Arnold, pp. 1–45.

Charlton, B. (2000) The new management of scientific knowledge in medicine: a change of direction with profound implications. In A. Miles, J. Hampton & B. Hurwitz (eds) *NICE, CHI and the NHS Reforms:*

Enabling Excellence or Imposing Control? London: Aesculapius Medical Press, pp. 13–32.

Classen, C. (1993) *Worlds of Sense: Exploring the Senses in History and Across Cultures*. London: Routledge.

Davies, C. (1999) *Reflexive Ethnography: A Guide to Researching Selves and Others*, London: Routledge.

Department of Health (2000) *Working Partnerships: Consumers in NHS Research*, 3rd Annual Report. London: HMSO.

Ellen, R. (1984) Introduction. In R. Ellen (ed.) *Ethnographic Research: A Guide to General Conduct*, Research Methods in Social Anthropology. London: Academic Press, pp. 1–12.

Farnell, B. (1994) Ethno-graphics and the moving body. *Man (NS)* **29**(4): 929–74.

Farnell, B. (2000) Getting out of the habitus: an alternative model of dynamically embodied social action. *Journal of the Royal Anthropological Institute* **6**(3): 397–418.

Foucault, M. (1973) *The Birth of the Clinic: An Archaeology of Medical Perception*. London: Tavistock Publications.

Frank, A. (1991) For a sociology of the body: an analytical review. In M. Featherstone, M. Hepworth & B. Turner (eds) *The Body: Social Process and Cultural Theory*. London: Sage, pp. 36–102.

Gregor, T. (1977) *Mehinaku: The Drama of Daily Life in a Brazilian Indian Village*. Chicago: University of Chicago Press.

Grosz, E. (1994) *Volatile Bodies: Toward a Corporeal Feminism*. Bloomington, IN: Indiana University Press.

Haug, F., Andresen, S., Bunz-Elfferding, A., Hauser, K., Lang, U., Laudan, M., Ludemann, M., Meir, U., Nemitz, B., Niehoff, E., Prinz, R., Rathzel, N., Scheu, M. & Thomas, C. (1987) *Female Sexualisation: A Collective Work of Memory*. London: Verso.

Herdt, G. (1990) *Intimate Communications: Erotics and the Study of Culture*. New York: Columbia University Press.

Hobart, M. (1993) Introduction: the growth of ignorance? In M. Hobart (ed.) *An Anthropological Critique of Development: The Growth of Ignorance*. London: Routledge, pp. 1–30.

Jackson, M. (1989) *Paths Towards a Clearing: Radical Empiricism and Ethnographic Inquiry*. Bloomington, IN: Indiana University Press.

Jay, M. (1999) Returning the gaze: the American response to the French critique of ocularcentrism. In G. Weiss & H. Fern Haber (eds) *Perspectives on Embodiment: The Intersections of Nature and Culture*. New York: Routledge, pp. 165–82.

Jenkins, R. (1992) *Pierre Bourdieu*. London: Routledge.

Jones, M. (1997) Thinking nursing. In S. Thorne & V. Hayes (eds)

Nursing Praxis: Knowledge and Action. Thousand Oaks, California: Sage, pp. 125–39.

Jorgensen, D. (1989) *Participant Observation: A Methodology for Human Studies*, Applied Social Research Methods Series, Vol. 15. Newbury Park, CA: Sage.

Lærke, A. (1998) By means of re-membering: notes on a fieldwork with English children. *Anthropology Today* **14**(1): 3–7.

Lawler, J. (1991) *Behind the Screens: Nursing, Somology and the Problem of the Body.* Melbourne: Churchill Livingstone.

Lawler, J. (ed.) (1997a) *The Body in Nursing.* South Melbourne: Churchill Livingstone.

Lawler, J. (1997b) Locating the body in nursing: an introduction. In J. Lawler (ed.) *The Body in Nursing.* South Melbourne: Churchill Livingstone, pp. 1–5.

Lawler, J. (1997c) Knowing the body and embodiment: methodologies, discourses and nursing. In J. Lawler (ed.) *The Body in Nursing.* South Melbourne: Churchill Livingstone, pp. 31–51.

Leder, D. (1990) *The Absent Body.* Chicago: University of Chicago Press.

Leder, D. (1992) *The Body in Medical Thought and Practice.* London: Kluwer Academic.

Lincoln, Y. & Denzin, N. (1994) The fifth moment. In N. Denzin & Y. Lincoln (eds) *Handbook of Qualitative Research.* Thousand Oaks, CA: Sage, pp. 575–86.

Loughlin, M. (2000) 'Quality' and 'excellence': meaning versus rhetoric. In A. Miles, J. Hampton & B. Hurwitz (eds) *NICE, CHI and the NHS Reforms: Enabling Excellence or Imposing Control?* London: Aesculapius Medical Press, pp. 1–12.

Menzies, I. (1970) *The Functioning of Social Systems as a Defence Against Anxiety* (reprint of Tavistock Pamphlet 3). London: Tavistock Institute.

Merleau-Ponty, M. (1962) *Phenomenology of Perception.* Evanston, IL: Northwestern University Press.

Okely, J. (1992) Anthropology and autobiography: participatory experience and embodied knowledge. In J. Okely & H. Callaway (eds) *Anthropology and Autobiography*, A.A. Monographs 29. London: Routledge, pp. 1–28.

Okely, J. (1994) Vicarious and sensory knowledge of chronology and change. In K. Hastup & P. Hervik (eds) *Social Experience and Anthropological Knowledge.* London: Routledge, pp. 45–64.

Parker, J. (1995) Searching for the body in nursing. In G. Gray and R. Pratt (eds) *Scholarship in the Discipline of Nursing.* Melbourne: Churchill Livingstone, pp. 333–54.

Pearson, A. (ed.) (1988) Primary nursing. In *Primary Nursing: Nursing in the Burford and Oxford Nursing Development Units*. London: Chapman & Hall, pp. 23–39.

Rock, P. (2001) Symbolic interactionism and ethnography. In P. Atkinson, A. Coffey, S. Delamont, J. Lofland & L. Lofland (eds) *Handbook of Ethnography*. London: Sage, pp. 26–38.

Rudberg, M. (1997) The researching body: the epistemophilic project. In K. Davis (ed.) *Embodied Practices: Feminist Perspectives on the Body*. London: Sage, pp. 182–201.

Rudge, T. (1996) Nursing wounds: exploring the presence of abjection in nursing practice. *Nursing Inquiry* 3(4): 250–51.

Sachs, A. (1990) *The Soft Vengeance of a Freedom Fighter*. London: Paladin.

Sartre, J.-P. (1984) *Being and Nothingness*. London: Methuen.

Savage, J. (1995) *Nursing Intimacy: An Ethnographic Approach to Nurse–Patient Interaction*. Harrow: Scutari.

Savage, J. (1997) Gestures of resistance: the nurse's body in contested space. *Nursing Inquiry* 7: 237–45.

Savage, J. (1999) Relative strangers: caring for patients as the expression of nurses' moral/political voice. In T. Kohn & R. McKechnie (eds) *Extending the Boundaries of Care: Medical Ethics and Caring Practices*. Oxford: Berg, pp. 181–201.

Savage, J. (2000) Participative observation: standing in the shoes of others? *Qualitative Health Research* **10**(3): 324–39.

Stoller, P. (1989) *The Taste of Ethnographic Things: The Senses in Anthropology*. Philadelphia: University of Pennsylvania Press.

Stoller, P. (1997) *Sensuous Scholarship*. Philadelphia: University of Pennsylvania Press.

Taussig, M. (1993) *Mimesis and Alterity: A Particular History of the Senses*. New York: Routledge.

Tonkin, E. (1984) Participant observation. In R.F. Ellen (ed.) *Ethnographic Research: A Guide to General Conduct*. London: Academic Press, pp. 213–23.

Young, I. (1990) Pregnant embodiment: subjectivity and alienation. In *Throwing Like a Girl and Other Essays in Feminist Philosophy and Social Theory*. Bloomington, IN: Indiana University Press, pp. 160–76.

CHAPTER 5

Self and others: the rigour and ethics of insider ethnography

Kate Gerrish

'I had felt somewhat uneasy about accompanying Judy (district nurse) on her visit to Karen (a single mother of two young children who had terminal breast cancer). It was surely going to be hard enough for Karen to talk to Dave, the clinical psychologist whom she was meeting with Judy for the first time, in order to start exploring how she might prepare her children for her impending death without having a researcher watching and listening to everything that was going on. What about my responsibility as a researcher to respect a participant's right to privacy? After all, I wasn't especially interested in how nurses provided care to dying patients.

Yet Judy had assured me before the visit that she had discussed my research with Karen, and Karen had confirmed to her that she was happy for me to join them. "Karen's expecting you, she'll think it strange if you don't turn up." Dave was also reported to have agreed to my presence. So I cast my doubts aside and went along... I talked through my research with both Karen and Dave and stressed that I would be happy to withdraw if they preferred, but both confirmed that I was welcome to stay...

When we got back in the car we sat in silence for a moment. I felt quite numbed by the emotional tension of the meeting. It was 12 years since I had worked as a sister on a haematology ward and encountered young women dying of cancer. Since moving into an academic post I had been cocooned from the emotional burden of caring. My coping mechanisms had been laid low and I felt quite vulnerable. Yet, I sensed that Judy had also found the visit difficult. She was the first to break the silence. "What do you think, Kate, from your experience, do you think we're going about it the right way? I'm so involved with Karen I find it hard to judge."

We spent the next half hour talking through the visit, reflecting on our observations, our feelings, how we thought the meeting had gone. I let Judy do most of the talking but shared something of my feelings – bearing in mind the circumstances I could hardly profess to be a dispassionate observer. And as I did so I became acutely aware of the tensions in my dual role as researcher and as nursing colleague. Our discussion provided extremely rich data on Judy's approach to providing individualised care, but at the same time I sensed that she was wanting and needing to use me as a colleague, someone who would listen to her concerns from a professional perspective. There was a sense of reciprocity in our relationship.'

The extract above is taken from field notes I made while I was engaged as a participant observer in an ethnographic study of district nursing practice. It highlights some of the complexity and messiness of undertaking research into nursing practice when the researcher is also a nurse. The extract raises a number of methodological and ethical questions about the kind of role nurse researchers should occupy in relation to research participants. Specifically,

- Should nurse researchers strive, on the one hand, to maintain distance from participants in order to enhance the objectivity (and thereby validity) of the data?
- On the other hand, is it legitimate for them to utilise their nursing expertise both as an active medium through which data are collected and subsequently interpreted, and as a means of reciprocating with participants?
- What are the implications for the credibility of the data when participants relate to them as nurses rather than as researchers?
- How should the ongoing consent of participants in a study be negotiated?
- On what basis can nurse researchers justify invading the private lives of participants at particularly vulnerable times in their lives?

It is important to note that there are no straightforward answers to these questions. Nurse researchers will respond differently depending upon the particular ontological and epistemological assumptions underpinning the methodologies they use. What is essential is that they are clear about such assumptions and can thereby justify their particular contribution to knowledge. Moreover, nurse researchers need to be explicit about how they interpret and apply methodologies that have their origins in the social sciences for use in a nursing context. Such action requires that they reflect with rigour on the decisions they make (as researchers and as nurses) and the consequences that arise from their actions.

My intention in writing this chapter is to illustrate how, as a nurse researcher, I have sought to address these issues in my own research. Specifically, I explore how the assumptions underpinning the particular ethnographic approach I adopted influenced my fieldwork. The study I refer to was concerned with exploring how the ideology of individualised care had been interpreted into nursing policy and had then been further modified in its implementation in practice. I was particularly interested in the implications for district nurses of providing individualised care to people from different ethnic backgrounds.

My interest in the topic had arisen from an earlier interview-based study (Gerrish *et al.*, 1996) in which I had been challenged by the apparent contradictions in the discourses of nurses as they described how they provided care to patients from different ethnic backgrounds. Although they claimed to practise individualised care, they also admitted difficulties in identifying and responding to the needs of minority ethnic patients because they lacked sufficient knowledge about cultural diversity or were inhibited by organisational constraints. Likewise, they spoke of the importance of treating patients as individuals yet expressed stereotypes of some minority ethnic communities. More perplexingly, some claimed to respond to individual needs yet at the same time asserted that they 'treated all patients the same'.

Reflecting upon the findings, I became anxious to try to unravel these apparent contradictions by finding out what was actually happening in practice as opposed to what nurses reported was taking place. I decided, therefore, to undertake a participant observational study of nursing practice. The decision to focus on district nurses, as opposed to hospital nurses, was made primarily on pragmatic grounds in that it would be easier to identify nurses who regularly provided care to patients from minority ethnic backgrounds in a community setting. In order to ensure that I had the opportunity to observe the care provided to patients from a range of different ethnic backgrounds I undertook periods of participant observation over a 12 month period with six district nursing teams employed by one community NHS trust. A more detailed account of the research can be found elsewhere (Gerrish, 1998, 1999, 2000, 2001).

The ethnographic approach

Put concisely, ethnography is a form of social research that relies on first hand knowledge of social processes, gathered *in situ* by the researcher:

> '... participating, overtly or covertly, in people's daily lives for an extended period of time, watching what happens, listening to what is said, asking questions – in fact, collecting whatever data are available to throw light on the issues that are the focus of the research.' (Hammersley & Atkinson, 1995: 1)

Although ethnography as an overall methodology is well established in nursing research even a cursory glance at the research literature will reveal various interpretations of ethnography. Some nurse researchers' use of ethnography is based on naturalistic assumptions (for example Mackenzie, 1992) in which the nurse as researcher seeks to study nursing phenomena in their natural setting objectively, endeavouring to distance him or herself from the participants who form the focus of the study. More recently there has been a developing critique of this traditional ethnographic approach that is informed by feminist, postmodern and post-structuralist debates about what constitutes an appropriate paradigm for researching nursing practice and developing nursing knowledge (see Bruni, 1995; Rudge, 1996; Cheek, 2000; Manias & Street, 2001). I do not propose to delve into these debates in detail but will summarise some of the main issues in so far as they contribute to locating my own position.

Naturalism adopts the position that in order to comprehend social reality the researcher needs to reveal the social world in a manner consistent with the participants' image of the world. The aim is 'to describe what happens in that setting, how the people involved see their own actions and those of others and the context in which the actions take place' (Hammersley & Atkinson, 1995: 6). It is based on the assumption that if the researcher is to understand social phenomena, he or she needs to discover the participants' definition of the situation, that is their perception and interpretation of reality and how these relate to their behaviour. Naturalists argue that the positivist's aspiration of discovering 'laws' of human behaviour is flawed since human behaviour is constructed and reconstructed on the basis of people's interpretations of the situations they encounter (Hammersley & Atkinson, 1995). It is only through accessing the meanings that people attribute to their own behaviour that the researcher can hope to understand social reality (Bryman, 1988).

However, in a similar vein to positivism, naturalism attempts to understand social phenomena as objects existing independently of the researcher who is seen as a potential source of bias that must be guarded against to preserve objectivity. The task of the ethnographer is to enter the field with as few preconceived ideas as possible in order to exert the minimum amount of influence on the nature of the data collected and its subsequent interpretation: in other words to become a 'professional stranger' (Agar, 1980). The philosophical position upon which naturalism's conception of objectivity is based is that of realism; the idea that the world has an existence independent of our perception of it, in other words whether or not we are aware of it or take an interest in it (Smith, 1983). Anti-realism stands in sharp contrast to realism and underpins postmodern and post-structural perspectives of social research. Rather than assuming that there is one reality that the researcher seeks to identify, anti-realists hold that there are multiple socially constructed realities that are devised by individuals as they attempt to make sense of their experiences (Guba & Lincoln, 1994).

The implications of adopting a realist or anti-realist ontology for the research enterprise become clearer when one considers the relationship between these ontologies and the theories of truth which they imply (Murphy et al., 1998). Realism is concerned with ascertaining a single truth, and is based on the assumption that direct and valid knowledge of reality is possible: that through our senses, we are able to perceive the world 'as it is' (Porter, 1993). By contrast, anti-realism holds that there can be no absolute truths. In recognising the plural nature of reality and the multiple positions from which it is possible to view aspects of reality, the researcher's account of the world is seen as one version amongst others (Cheek, 2000). Moreover, it is recognised that any attempt to gain insight into the inner life of another individual or group is inevitably filtered through the researcher's language, gender, social class and ethnicity. To this end, there are no truly objective observations of social reality, rather observations that are socially situated in the worlds of the observer and the observed (Denzin & Lincoln, 1994).

It is not the intention here to debate the arguments for or against these two ontological positions but rather to clarify how I have resolved the challenges that each one raises in my own research. I have been influenced by Hammersley (1992) who, in arguing the case for what he terms 'subtle realism', proposes an approach to ethnography that straddles both naturalistic and postmodern imperatives. Porter (1996) outlines the benefits for nurse researchers of adopting a similar hybrid position, that of 'critical realist' ethnography.

Subtle realism, according to Hammersley (1992), rejects the notion that it is possible to have certainty about claims to knowledge. Rather, in recognising that knowledge is provisional, the objective should be the search for knowledge about which we can be reasonably confident. Such confidence is based upon judgements about the credibility and plausibility of knowledge claims. Phenomena are deemed to exist independently of the researcher's claims about them and these claims may be more or less accurate. The aim of social research from this perspective is to represent reality, and any given reality can be represented from a range of different perspectives. This opens up the possibility of multiple, valid descriptions of the same phenomenon. Such representations inevitably reflect the assumptions that researchers bring to the research and rather than engaging in futile attempts to eliminate the effects of the researcher, it is recognised that researchers are part of the social world they study and through a reflexive approach attempts are made to try to understand these effects and how their values and interests may impinge upon the research.

Having outlined my interpretation of ethnographic method-ology, I propose to reflect upon the implications of this stance in relation to some of the methodological and ethical issues associated with my role as both participant (nurse) and observer (researcher).

The nurse as participant observer

Nurse researchers who seek through participant observation to study nursing practice are in a unique and privileged position. Their parallel status as researcher and nurse can assist them in gaining access to the research setting and in establishing rapport with the research participants, be they patients or nurses. Moreover, the insights they already have into the social world of nursing can be used to inform their data collection. However, the very advantages that dual status brings can also prove problematic. It may be dif-ficult both for nurse researchers and for research participants to differentiate clearly between the two aspects of the role, and relationships may be built and disclosures made on the basis of being perceived as a nurse rather than a researcher. Nurse researchers may also find it difficult to distance themselves suffi-ciently from the values and beliefs that underpin their own pro-fessional practice in order to understand the social world of those who form the focus of their study. Wrestling with these tensions became an integral part of my own experiences.

One of the greatest challenges for the participant observer is that of living simultaneously in two worlds, that of participation and that of research. Hammersley and Atkinson (1995: 113) describe the situation thus:

> 'While ethnographers may adopt a variety of roles, the usual aim throughout is to maintain a more or less marginal posi-tion, thereby providing access to participant perspectives but at the same time minimising the dangers of over-rapport.'

Maintaining ones' position on the margins is not easy.

My role during fieldwork was first and foremost that of a researcher but I used my nursing expertise to assist and inform my data collection. I chose to present myself as a qualified nurse; I wore a staff nurse's uniform and assisted, as appropriate, in caregiving. I had not worked as a district nurse for some years, and although this caused some personal anxiety as initially I lacked confidence in a clinical context, it had its advantages. I was able to exploit my position as a 'returning nurse' in pursuit of my research objectives. It was legitimate for me to ask the naive questions that would not normally be expected of a competent qualified practitioner. These were precisely the questions that I needed to ask as a participant observer in order to explore the cultural assumptions underpinning the nurses' practices.

However, as a nurse researching nursing practice I became only too aware of the tensions between the *objectivity* of observation as a researcher and the *subjectivity* of participation as a nurse. Hammersley and Atkinson (1995) highlight this tension between acting competently while at the same time privately struggling to suspend for analytical purposes precisely those assumptions that are taken for granted in relations with participants. The challenge lies in trying to balance involvement with detachment, familiarity with strangeness, and closeness with distance (Adler & Adler, 1994). However, such manoeuvring was not easy. As the earlier extract from fieldwork cited at the beginning of this chapter implies, it was difficult to distance myself from my emotional response (as a fellow human being and as a nurse) to Karen's predicament in order to observe as a researcher.

Moreover, in recognising that my own assumptions reflected the dominant professional ideologies of the nurses whom I studied, it was a constant struggle to maintain sufficient distance in order to treat these assumptions as problematic. Yet achieving such distance was essential, especially in view of my focus on ethnicity. I was aware of the criticisms levied at nursing in respect of its ethnocentric professional ideologies and practices (Stokes, 1991). Moreover, I realised from the outset that for a white nurse researcher to study the provision of nursing care to patients from minority ethnic backgrounds was something of a high-risk enterprise. Criticism has been levied at white researchers for working within an ethnocentric framework that imposes a particular interpretation on the collection and analysis of data. Ethnocentric biases are seen to inhibit an understanding of the social world from the perspectives of members of some minority ethnic communities whose experiences of oppression have shaped their lives in a way that is difficult for white researchers to appreciate (Stanfield II, 1993; Kelleher, 1996). I endeavoured, therefore, constantly to question my own assumptions and interpretations of the data through my engagement with the literature, discussions with colleagues and by intermittently taking time out of the field to reflect.

Such blurring of boundaries between researcher and nurse was also evident in the ways in which both nurses and patients responded to me. Although I sought to be open about my role as a researcher, I sensed that there were occasions when both nurses and patients expected me to respond as a nurse. As the earlier extract from fieldwork illustrates, sometimes the nurses sought my views on their approach to care. In such situations it seemed wholly inappropriate not to respond. The nurses had judged (correctly) that I would hold a professional opinion about the particular situation. Nevertheless, rather than foreground my own nursing expertise, I endeavoured to use the opportunity to encourage the nurses to reflect upon their own position.

There were also occasions when I found myself alone with patients for substantial periods of time while the nurse took the opportunity to talk in private with the carers. In such situations, although patients were aware of my presence as a researcher, they also responded to me as a nurse, often volunteering intimate details regarding their medical and social history or seeking my professional advice on matters of concern. I found it difficult to adopt a non-interventionist stance given the circumstances. However, the boundaries between what might be considered data gained with the consent of the person concerned and disclosures made in response to me as a 'nurse' were unclear.

In adopting a subtle realist perspective I had accepted as inevitable the fact that I would exert some influence on the research setting and the behaviour of participants. Yet it was difficult to gauge the extent of this effect. The nurses themselves reported that, from their perspective, my presence had not affected the relationship they had with patients and carers, although I did not seek the views of patients. The nurses did, however, make me aware of instances in which my probing had challenged them to question aspects of their own practice, and in some cases this had acted as a catalyst to introducing change.

Linked to the unintended effects that I might exert on the research setting was the related issue of whether I should deliberately offer the benefits of my own expertise to the nurses. Atkinson and Hammersley (1994) suggest that researchers may legitimately trade on their personal expertise in terms of their knowledge and resources in order to gain access to the research setting. Moreover, they highlight the benefits of demonstrating that the researcher is not an exploitive interloper but has something to give in return. Such reciprocity took various forms: the essential second pair of hands to assist in caregiving; a professional companion who stimulated them to think more deeply about their practice; and a colleague who provided moral support in difficult situations.

Adopting a subtle realist perspective also made me aware of the need to take into account the personal, social and cultural identities of both the researcher and the researched. One of the methodological challenges of researching ethnicity is that participants will respond in ways they consider appropriate in the context of how they perceive the ethnic identity of the researcher in relation to their own identity (Andersen, 1993). That I was a white female researcher examining how white female nurses provided care to patients from minority ethnic backgrounds inevitably influenced the nature of the data I collected and the subsequent interpretations I placed on the data. The nurses related to me as 'one of them' in their accounts of caring for minority ethnic patients. This appeared to be a reflection not only of my status as a nurse, but also of their perception of my ethnicity. Had I been, in their eyes, from a visible minority ethnic background, they and their patients may well have responded to me differently.

Ethical principles translated into practice

The complex and changing nature of field relationships together with the shifting composition of people who interact with the main participants require the nurse researcher to resolve ethical dilemmas on a day-to-day basis. Although there are ethical principles such as informed consent, respecting the rights of participants to confidentiality, anonymity, privacy and protection from harm, there is no blueprint as to how these principles should be interpreted in practice. Rather, it is left to researchers to act in an ethically acceptable manner, taking due account of the research objectives, the situation in which the research is being undertaken, and the values and interests of the people involved. In the end, the ethical decisions nurse researchers make are a matter of judgement and open to challenge.

The very nature of ethnographic research raises a number of issues regarding how consent is gained from participants. Although it is generally agreed that participants should be informed about the study in a comprehensive way and consent freely to be studied, the notion of informed consent in overt participant observation is highly complex. First, the researcher has to decide from whom consent should be sought. Clearly, it is appropriate to gain consent from the participants who form the focus of the study, in my case members of the district nursing teams. Additionally, although I was not seeking information from patients directly, I still considered it important to gain the patients' agreement to my observing their care. However, deciding on an appropriate means of gaining such consent was not easy. I was sensitive to the power invested in my position as a researcher in relation to participants in general, and patients in particular, who were vulnerable by virtue of their need for nursing care. At the same time I needed to take into account the power relationships between the nurses and their patients. In negotiating with the nurses to ask the patients' permission on my behalf, ideally in advance of our visit, I reasoned that patients might feel more able to refuse the request if it did not come directly from me and, indeed, there were a few instances where patients expressed a preference for me not to visit. However, it was impossible to judge whether the fact that the majority of patients consented to my observing their care was the result of a genuine willingness on their part to participate in the research or the result of compliance with the request of a health professional on whose future care they were dependent. Moreover, the fact that the study took place in a natural setting meant that I had little control over who entered the field. In addition to the nurses and their patients, there were numerous other people who, while not the main actors, became the supporting cast in helping me gain an understanding of nursing practice. Whenever the opportunity arose, I introduced myself as a nurse researcher and explained the purpose of the study; however, it was impractical to gain fully informed consent from everyone who was involved tangentially in the study.

Second, questions arise regarding what 'fully informed' might mean in situations where the research design evolves during the course of the study (Murphy *et al.*, 1998). Research questions are fairly tentative at the beginning of fieldwork, and it is through progressive focusing and theoretical sampling that the specifics of the study are negotiated (Hammersley & Atkinson, 1995). For this reason, it is rarely possible to gain fully informed consent in advance of fieldwork. Rather, at the time of negotiating initial entry into the setting, I needed to make clear to the nurses the emergent nature of the research design and then engage in ongoing negotiations about what I observed over time. It was also important to acknowledge the autonomy of the research participants and to be prepared to withdraw or amend the emergent design in the light of participants' wishes (Murphy *et al.*, 1998). In this regard I had indicated to the nurses that although I was keen to accompany them throughout the working day, if there were situations where they considered my participation inappropriate, then I would withdraw. In the event, there were a few occasions where the nurses exercised this discretion.

Although one of the greatest strengths of participant observation is its unobtrusiveness, it is this very strength that renders it liable to abuse in respect of the invasion of privacy. Invasion of privacy may take two forms; venturing into *private places* and *misrepresenting oneself as a member* (Adler & Adler, 1994). By undertaking domiciliary visits, I was seeking not only to observe the privacy of the nurse–patient interaction, but also to do so in a private setting in which I had no right of access either as a nurse or as a researcher. The excerpt from my field notes at the beginning of this chapter illustrates the unease I experienced between my desire as a researcher to observe the full diversity of nursing practice and my professional values to uphold the privacy and dignity of vulnerable patients. Even when I had gained consent from participants, I did not consider that I had an automatic right to accompany the nurses. Rather, I discussed the particular circumstances with the nurses before making a decision.

The point about misrepresenting oneself as a member is also pertinent. As indicated earlier, there were occasions when I perceived that nurses and patients responded to me as a nurse rather than a researcher. My appearance in a nurse's uniform no doubt exacerbated this. Such misrepresentation, albeit unintentional, has implications for data collection. Finch (1984) cautions that in indepth interviewing where both interviewer and interviewee are women, material that is highly personal may be elicited in what is seemingly a friendly relationship and with what she suggests may be very flimsy guarantees of confidentiality. Nurse researchers, by virtue of their perceived professional standing, are in a similar position to elicit intimate information from both health care professionals and patients, information that participants might choose not to disclose to a non-nurse researcher. Although nurse researchers may undertake to maintain the anonymity of the individual participants, they have little influence over how the findings will be used once they are in the public domain. In recognising that knowledge represents power and such power may be used to manipulate those who are relatively powerless, Finch warns that it is not only individual interests but also the collective interests of the group under study that may be compromised. Nurse researchers need, therefore, to give due consideration to the unintended as well as the intended consequences of their research.

The thorny issue of intervention

During the course of fieldwork, nurse researchers may well observe situations that they see as requiring some form of clinical intervention. The question then arises as to whether they should intervene. However, taking action to remedy the situation will challenge the researcher's status as a neutral observer by transgressing the researcher–participant boundary and may well raise ethical dilemmas in relation to the research itself (Rudge, 1995). Fontana and Frey (1994) advise that the researcher's moral responsibility towards the participants should, if necessary, override the interests of the study. However, in the case of ethnographic research the participants are frequently not a homogeneous group and the concerns of one group may be at variance with those of others.

Conflict can then arise between the researcher's loyalty to those studied and the wider responsibility to reveal practices deemed to be against the interests of a vulnerable group within a setting (Murphy *et al.*, 1998). The researcher may well find him or herself in possession of information or observe unethical or rule-breaking behaviour which could harm the interests of some participants if revealed. The difficulty arises if those in authority who grant access to the research setting expect the researcher to report such behaviour (Burgess, 1985). Such tensions can be compounded where the researcher is occupying a position that carries with it particular professional responsibilities. Whereas the code of professional conduct (United Kingdom Central Council, 1992) charges nurses with the responsibility to act in such a manner as to promote and safeguard the interests and well-being of patients, it is difficult to interpret the code in a research context (Johnson, 1993).

Throughout fieldwork I was acutely aware of the dissonance between my responsibilities as a nurse towards patients should I observe nursing practice that I considered detrimental to their well-being, and the effect I would have on the research should I challenge a particular nurse's practice. I had decided that as a general policy if I witnessed anything that I considered resembled grossly unsafe or negligent practice then I would compromise my position as a researcher and intervene in the patient's interests. Fortunately, such situations did not arise. However, what I did encounter much more frequently were instances where practice was not particularly bad but perhaps could have been better. There was no easy way to resolve these concerns as each situation was different. In the end I exercised my professional discretion in deciding whether to intervene. Where I judged the behaviour not to be particularly detrimental to the patient's well-being, I remained silent. However, I did intercede on a few occasions where I was particularly concerned that a patient might be disadvantaged. For example, in a situation where I suspected that a young South Asian man who was interpreting for his elderly grandmother who did not speak English had not fully understood the instructions provided by the nurse concerning analgesic medication, I deliberately joined in the conversation to seek clarification of his understanding and create the opportunity for the nurse to provide further explanation. I was aware that the nurse might interpret such actions as criticisms of her practice. However, the fact that I frequently participated in conversations between nurses and their patients meant that it was not too difficult to intervene tactfully. Although there was a risk of compromising the research by affecting adversely the relationship I had developed with the nurse, I decided that my professional accountability took precedence.

Conclusion

Having focused on the particulars of my own research, what are the wider implications that can be drawn out? First, it is important that nurse researchers give serious consideration to the methodologies they use and in particular, to the ontological and epistemological assumptions that underpin these methodologies. It is not sufficient to say that one is using an ethnographic approach. As I have pointed out, there is a range of ontological and epistemological assumptions that researchers may draw upon in interpreting ethnographic methodology and in order that nurse researchers can justify the claims they make regarding their particular contribution to nursing knowledge they need to make their position explicit. From a subtle realist perspective, it is recognised that although as researchers we search for truth, we will never grasp the whole truth. Nevertheless, we strive through rigour and integrity to move closer to a more valid understanding of the truth of a situation.

It is also essential that nurse researchers reflect with rigour on their location as researchers and as nurses in the research setting. It is unrealistic to assume that nurse researchers can enter the field as a *tabula rasa*. Rather than regard their personal, social and cultural identities as a source of bias that must be guarded against in order to maintain objectivity, nurse researchers need to try to understand how these may impinge upon their research. However, nurse researchers also need to consider carefully the extent to which they foreground their nursing expertise. Although such expertise can be used with great effect throughout fieldwork, unless they recognise and challenge their own taken-for-granted assumptions which reflect the dominant professional ideologies, they may fail to recognise the significance of data which cuts across these assumptions.

As nurses as well as researchers, nurse researchers should consider how the ethics of nursing practice interact with the ethics of research practice. Where nurses make explicit use of their professional background as a medium to facilitate data collection, they are professionally accountable for their nursing as well as their research conduct. Ethical dilemmas are never easy to resolve; however, what is essential is that nurse researchers explain the rationale behind the decisions they make in order that the wider academic and professional community can form some reasoned opinion about their conduct.

Finally, in recognising the complexity and messiness of researching the social world of nursing, nurse researchers need to explain how they have adapted methodologies drawn from the social sciences for use in a nursing context. In doing so, they should not be daunted by the apparent lack of purity in methods, but rather, as Johnson *et al.* (2001) suggest, they should accept this reality while maintaining rigour through integrity, reflexivity, clear accounts of their methods and a constructive critique of their work.

References

Adler, P.A. & Adler, P. (1994) Observational techniques. In N.K. Denzin & Y.S. Lincoln (eds) *Handbook of Qualitative Research*. Thousand Oaks, CA: Sage, pp. 377–92.

Agar, M.H. (1980) *The Professional Stranger: An Informal Introduction to Ethnography*. New York: Academic Press.

Andersen, M.L. (1993) Studying across difference: race, class and gender in qualitative research. In J.H. Stanfield II & R.M. Dennis (eds) *Race and Ethnicity in Research Methods*. Newbury Park, CA: Sage, pp. 39–52.

Atkinson, P. & Hammersley, M. (1994) Ethnography and participant observation. In N.K. Denzin & Y.S. Lincoln (eds) *Handbook of Qualitative Research*. Thousand Oaks, CA: Sage, pp. 248–61.

Bruni, N. (1995) Reshaping ethnography: contemporary postpositivist possibilities. *Nursing Inquiry* 2: 44–52.

Bryman, A. (1988) *Quantity and Quality in Social Research*. London: Routledge.

Burgess, R. (1985) The whole truth? Some ethical problems of research in a comprehensive school. In R.G. Burgess (ed.) *Strategies of Educational Research: Qualitative Methods*. Lewes: Falmer Press, pp. 141–62.

Cheek, J. (2000) *Postmodern and Poststructural Approaches to Nursing Research*. Thousand Oaks, CA: Sage.

Denzin, N.K. & Lincoln, Y.S. (1994) Introduction: entering the field of qualitative research. In N.K. Denzin & Y.S. Lincoln (eds) *Handbook of Qualitative Research*. Thousand Oaks, CA: Sage, pp. 1–17.

Finch, J. (1984) 'It's great to have someone to talk to': the ethics and politics of interviewing women. In C. Bell & H. Roberts (eds) *Social Researching: Policies, Problems and Practice*. London: Routledge & Kegan Paul, pp. 70–85.

Fontana, A. & Frey, J.H. (1994) Interviewing: the art of science. In N.K. Denzin & Y.S. Lincoln (eds) *Handbook of Qualitative Research*. Thousand Oaks, CA: Sage, pp. 361–76.

Gerrish, C.A. (1998) The provision of individualised care in a multi-ethnic society: an ethnographic study of nursing policy and practice. PhD dissertation, University of Nottingham, England.

Gerrish, K. (1999) Inequalities in service provision: an examination of institutional influences on the provision of district nursing care to minority ethnic communities. *Journal of Advanced Nursing* 30: 1263–71.

Gerrish, K. (2000) Individualised care: its conceptualisation and practice within a multi-ethnic society. *Journal of Advanced Nursing* 32: 91–9.

Gerrish, K. (2001) The nature and effect of communication difficulties arising from interactions between district nurses and South Asian patients and their carers. *Journal of Advanced Nursing* 33: 566–74.

Gerrish, K., Husband, C. & Mackenzie, J. (1996) *Nursing for a Multi-ethnic Society*. Buckingham: Open University Press.

Guba, E.G. & Lincoln, Y.S. (1994) Competing paradigms in qualitative research. In N.K. Denzin & Y.S. Lincoln (eds) *Handbook of Qualitative Research*. Thousand Oaks, CA: Sage, pp. 105–17.

Hammersley, M. (1992) Ethnography and realism. In M. Hammersley (ed.) *What's Wrong with Ethnography?* London: Routledge, pp. 43–56.

Hammersley, M. & Atkinson, P. (1995) *Ethnography: Principles and Practice*, 2nd edn. London: Routledge.

Johnson, M. (1993) Unpopular patients reconsidered: an interpretative ethnography of the process of social judgement in a hospital ward. PhD dissertation, University of Manchester, England.

Johnson, M., Long, T. & White, A. (2001) Arguments for 'British Pluralism' in qualitative research. *Journal of Advanced Nursing* 33: 243–9.

Kelleher, D. (1996) A defence of the use of the terms 'ethnicity' and 'culture'. In D. Kelleher & S. Hillier (eds) *Researching Cultural Differences in Health*. London: Routledge, pp. 69–90.

Mackenzie, A. (1992) Learning from experience in the community: an ethnographic study of district nurse students. PhD dissertation, University of Surrey, England.

Manias, E. & Street, A. (2001) Rethinking ethnography: reconstructing nursing relationships. *Journal of Advanced Nursing* **33**: 234–42.

Murphy, E., Dingwall, R., Greatbatch, D., Parker, S. & Watson, P. (1998) Qualitative research methods in health technology assessment: a review of the literature. *Health Technology Assessment* **2** (16).

Porter, S. (1993) Nursing research conventions: objectivity or obfuscation? *Journal of Advanced Nursing* **18**: 137–43.

Porter, S. (1996) Breaking the boundaries between nursing and sociology: a critical realist ethnography of the theory practice gap. *Journal of Advanced Nursing* **24**: 413–20.

Rudge, T. (1995) Response: Insider ethnography: researching nursing from within. *Nursing Inquiry* **2**: 58.

Rudge, T. (1996) (Re)writing ethnography: the unsettling questions for nursing research raised by post-structural approached to 'the field'. *Nursing Inquiry* **3**: 146–52.

Smith, J. (1983) Quantitative versus qualitative research: an attempt to clarify the issue. *Educational Researcher* **12**: 6–13.

Stanfield II, J.H. (1993) Epistemological considerations. In J.H. Stanfield II & R.M. Dennis (eds) *Race and Ethnicity in Research Methods*. Newbury Park, CA: Sage, pp. 16–36.

Stokes, G. (1991) A transcultural nurse is about. *Senior Nurse* **11** (1): 40–42.

United Kingdom Central Council (1992) *Code of Professional Conduct*. London: UKCC.

Stories

The chapters in Part III explore how to draw upon the stories that nurses and patients tell to enhance knowledge of nursing practice and of patients' methods for dealing with health and illness.

While there has been an explosion of interest in narrative within the medical field in the past decade, the authors in this part argue that this interest is largely under-theorised and, as a consequence, of limited use. In contrast, these chapters present methodological approaches which treat stories as one of the ways in which the field of nursing practice and the experience of illness is made up, that is as both topic and resource.

The authors also present methods for drawing on specific theoretical perspectives to analyse and make sense of patients' and nurses' narratives. Specifically, the authors show how the choice and development of a method and analytical framework can be congruent with, rather than intrusive upon, the narrative genre deployed by the subjects of research as 'authors' of their own identity.

CHAPTER 6

Researching story and narrative in nursing: an object-relations approach

Judith M. Parker & John Wiltshire

The scope and dimensions of nursing practices, and the ways in which patients deal with their experiences of health and illness, are often communicated in stories. However, it was not until recently that stories were considered appropriate material for research. As Sandelowski (1991) pointed out, it was only in the context of the shift away from positivism and towards interpretation in the behavioural and social sciences that attention in research endeavours began to be paid to the narrative nature of human beings. As a consequence there has been an explosion of interest in narrative within the health field in general over the past decade or so. The work of Kleinman (1988), Hunter (1991) and Frank (1995), in particular, has stimulated a widespread focus on the contribution that stories can make to our understanding of medical experience. Not surprisingly, this interest has spread to nursing, and notions of narrative and story are now being drawn upon in a number of ways in nursing practice and research.

Increasingly, narrative is being understood in nursing practice in therapeutic terms. The 'restorying' of profound life experience is a technique to facilitate greater acceptance of what has happened (Sandelowski, 1994; Canales, 1997; Clark and Standard, 1997; McLeod, 1997; Moules and Amundson, 1997), and as a professional development tool for nurses to facilitate a deeper understanding of self and others (Bowles, 1995). There is similar interest in story and narrative within nursing research, and Sandelowski (1991) has been a significant figure in identifying the scope of narrative approaches and methods of analysis for qualitative research in nursing.

In the burgeoning literature on narrative research that has

appeared over the past decade, a considerable amount draws upon phenomenological–hermeneutic method (e.g. Benner, 1991; Tanner *et al.*, 1993; Darbyshire, 1994; Nehls, 1995) and humanistic philosophy (e.g. Svedlund *et al.*, 1999). Other researchers take an atheoretical and somewhat methodologically naive approach to narrative which nevertheless identifies important material about people's everyday understanding about disease and likely responses (e.g. Facione and Giancarlo, 1998). Some researchers are drawing upon narrative data to offer a feminist critique of aspects of health care (e.g. Stevens, 1996). The so-called postmodern turn has resulted in notions of a relational narrative and its relevance for nursing knowledge (Gadow, 1995), nursing ethics (Gadow, 1999) and establishing dialogue necessary for cultural pluralism in nursing and health care (Sakalys, 2000).

More recently, researchers writing from a post-structuralist perspective have pointed out problems in these approaches to narrative research. Crowe (1998), for example, questions assumptions about the construction of subjectivity in the process of data collection that underpins qualitative research methodologies. She argues that the notions that reality can be apprehended by capturing the individual's point of view and that qualitative researchers can directly represent lived experience in language are ideologically based assumptions that need to be challenged. Harden (2000) supports this position in calling for a less naive understanding of the complexities of the language with which the individual speaks, and argues that the emphasis placed on seeking an authentic story of the life of the research subject is misguided. Similar critiques have come from writers such as Atkinson and Silverman (1997), pointing to the need to correct 'uncritical, neo-romantic celebrations of the speaking subject' (p. 305) and the celebration of 'the interview and the narrative data it produces as an especially authentic mode of social representation' (p. 312). They go on to suggest that life narratives are 'always pastiche pieced together, always changeable and fallible' (p. 319).

We have sought to work with story and narrative in a way which takes account of these postmodern critiques of subjectivity and language, but our approach is not specifically post-structural. Our critique of post-structuralism stems from our view that it does not permit analysis of or provide insight into pre-lingual or alingual aspects of experience. Our reason for working with psychoanalytic concepts lies in our understanding that there are aspects of nursing practice flowing from the body that cannot be spoken, but must, nevertheless, be dealt with. We draw upon one key aspect of psychoanalytic object-relations theory as an organising framework; this is the notion of 'containing' first advanced by Bion (1961). We have brought this concept to bear in the understanding of two sets of practices within nursing – the traditional end-of-shift handover and the nursing management of stoma – to outline a methodological and theoretically informed approach to analysis of nurses' and patients' stories. We examine how story and narrative function to contain and make manageable disturbing emotions that arise in the course of everyday nursing practice and in the savage assaults on identity and self-image that often form part of the experience of being a patient.

In our work we recognise story-telling as an important feature of nursing experience. We achieve rigour and validity through applying some key psychoanalytic concepts to the multiplicity of evidence. In this way raw events and unprocessed stories are converted into useable terms and concepts to further the advancement of nursing knowledge. Critically, research findings such as those on the handover and the work of stomal therapy nurses, can help to substantiate the efficacy of aspects of nursing practice whose rationality is normally invisible, and which nurses may find difficult to justify in the face of efficiency drives. This is their critical and political contribution to nursing knowledge.

Story and narrative

It is helpful to think about the terms 'story' and 'narrative' and to see whether or not some distinctions can be made between them (Wiltshire, 1995). A first step in analysis is to refuse to take these terms for granted. As a survey of the literature will indicate, these words are often used interchangeably. Sometimes, 'story' is used to mean little more than 'account'. At one level, everything, including science, is a 'story', and what is meant by this is more or less any cognitive response to the life-world. 'Story' is not always honorific or benign. When a patient was undergoing an eye test, and gave inconsistent results, the optometrist responded, roughly, 'you keep changing your story'. (And this is a story, too.) Clearly, 'story' needs to be thought about.

To begin with, it may be helpful to reserve the term 'story' for verbal communications. When a researcher cites a patient's story, then, it would be understood that she is referring to something told to her, and recorded by her. Accepting this simple step involves some important consequences. A story is necessarily contingent: it is produced in the matrix between two persons, on a particular occasion. A person's 'story' (their account, their testimony) may well vary when they tell it to another person, or on another occasion. This is not necessarily to relegate story to an inferior category of evidence to narrative, but it will be helpful if 'narrative' is understood as a more complex product than story. Narrative is more closely associated than story with formality, reflection and organisation. A narrative is not simply one thing after another – that is a chronicle – but a communication in which relations are found between the things that are recalled or represented. This means that the construction of a narrative often involves reflection upon the material.

'Narrative' is more readily associated than 'story' with formal publication (but think of the 'short story'). The point to emphasise is that narrative tends to imply some degree of removal, of detachment from the original experience. One might put this clearly by saying that the nurse researcher collects 'stories', but that she shapes these into a 'narrative'. The shaping involves reflection on the material, bringing to the material a conceptual structure not necessarily found within it, and usually the presence of something approaching an ethical element. This is why the usage of 'narrative' is generally honorific or respectful: it does not have the slightly tentative or confabulated quality that the word 'story' carries.

These distinctions are, of course, oversimple. They are intended only as tools, and as a way to clarify the field. One would not wish to derogate a patient's story, or to assume that written testimony is necessarily more valuable than verbal. Many people can express themselves vividly and meaningfully through the spoken word, and do not reflect much upon their experience. But it is the province of the narrator, and of narrative, we suggest, to do so. In his book *The Wounded Storyteller*, Arthur Frank (1995) refers to the 'chaos narrative'. Frank seeks by this term to indicate the absence of apparent meaning or coherence in lives dominated by chronic neurological illness, but his use of the word 'narrative' here confuses the issues. A narrative cannot meaningfully refer to a mere sequence of real-life events. A literary term, it refers necessarily to a form of expression. 'Chaos narrative' strains language to the point of paradox. In Frank's defence, one might say that the extremity of the experiences he refers to seem to license this stretching or distortion of language to reflect them.

Narrative, then, normally involves the uncovering or creation of meaning within experience. This makes it analogous to the enterprise that the nurse researcher is embarked upon. The researcher's narrative, itself no doubt including many stories, will involve reflection upon the material collected. Order or meaning will be discerned within or imputed to the research material – and often this will be through the discernment of common or analogous elements across a range of discrete contributions. But while the production of a research paper or thesis is a solitary and individual experience, the material to be dealt with will be produced as a collaboration between two or more human beings. The researcher needs to bear in mind always that the narrative she is producing has to reflect, perhaps even to honour, the story-like quality of the primary human material. It is this tension that is the biggest challenge in researching story and narrative.

Confronting the data

If we take our own experience as an example, the least of your problems as a nursing researcher will be the gathering of interesting material. Whatever the subject of research, it will almost certainly involve your presence at and recording of nursing practice. This attendance at handover meetings, interviews with patients, focus groups, etc., will produce great amounts of interesting material. It will be arresting, perturbing, fascinating, appalling, moving; it will include stories of human ingenuity, iniquity, comedy, suffering. It will seem richer, more thought-provoking, more immediate and more relevant than a novel or short story. Having collected it, you will feel that it demands to be told, to be circulated, to be known.

But you are committed to research. What you produce out of this mass of dramatic material must be a 'contribution to knowledge' – must be, at the very least, an argument. If you have a grant, or are writing a thesis, then you will be expected to produce 'results'. You cannot simply reproduce this material, even if that were possible. Besides, reproduction is impossible. Even if you decide that you want to reproduce it, you will inevitably select, edit, reword: what you make of the stories you have attended to will be different from what your participants told you. (It might be best directly to embrace fiction or poetry as your mode of response, and many researchers interested in working with this kind of material have in fact done this.)

But let us say that you choose not to take this route. You do not want simply to pay tribute to the stories of courage and suffering and mishap and stoicism you have heard. You want to produce something helpful, something that may just make the lives of your participants and similar patients easier, something that speaks to the experiences of staff and provides insight into aspects of their relationships with patients: something that is useful. Your task is to process this material so that something new and interesting may come out of it. You accept then, from the start, that you are not simply a 'witness' of what you have been told, that you are a commentator, an interpreter. Nor are you solely an 'advocate' of the patient (though that may be part of your motivation): you are committed by the very project to a different field: to the production of research-based knowledge.

It is important not to underestimate the challenge and the momentousness of what you face. The production of tangible results out of qualitative research material is not easy. In some ways the difficulty you face is comparable to the challenge faced by the first scientists or 'natural philosophers' when they began to study the physical world, and which they resolved by breaking down into smaller components. There are many pressures on qualitative nurse researchers to imagine that the form of work they produce must be analogous to medical science, that results must be 'objective', reproducible, verifiable, and must contribute to quantifiable health outcomes. Despite the rise of interpretative and critical approaches to research in nursing and the arguments produced identifying the ways in which qualitative research differs from a medical scientific approach, the pressures continue and the arguments still appear to need making.

In our research we were quite clear that we needed to be aware of the historical and social basis of our material, that it constantly changes and is responsive to many pressures. We were also quite clear that we were not studying an organism, a body, conceived as essentially separate from the rest of the world, isolated conceptually for the purposes of study. We were focusing not on the body of the patient, but the patient, a person, a selfhood, who exists in relationship to other persons, other selfhoods. Additionally, we recognised that human beings tend to understand the world and to express themselves not rationally but symbolically. We were dealing with an interactive and psychological world that does not obey the same laws as the physical world. This is why we felt it was necessary to locate our study within a conceptualisation of the nature of interpersonal relationships.

Object-relations theory

We found psychoanalytic thought, specifically one key aspect of object-relations theory, helpful in understanding and organizing the primary material we collected. This is the notion, first advanced by W.R. Bion (1961) of 'containing'. All object-relations theorists owe their basic focus to Melanie Klein (1935) and the emphasis in her work on the infant's conflicted and divided impulses towards its mother. In her work, Freud's (1912) discovery of the 'transference' becomes crucial, and this makes it an especially fruitful source for thinking not about the isolated, individual psyche upon whose inner life Freud concentrated, but upon that psyche's relation to others – to the 'objects' of the group's informal name. In other words, object-relations is a theory or conceptual tool which seeks to make sense of the conscious as well as the unconscious flows of feeling that form what we call a relationship between two or more persons, and often between mother and child.

We have found that object-relations psychoanalytic thought has an especial pertinancy and usefulness to the understanding of nursing experience. First, psychoanalysis is a discourse which has evolved terms to describe relationships. Object-relations psychoanalysis is particularly fruitful in concepts which address the particular relationship patterns that develop between the professional, the analyst, and his or her patient. It therefore offers a number of concepts with which to address those analogous (though very different) relationships between professional and patient which makes up key parts of nursing experience.

Second, psychoanalytic writers have come to terms with the earliest experiences of the infant psyche. Unable to think, subject to sensations of both gratification and frustration which are overwhelming, the child in its earliest days of life is the vehicle of feelings of an intensity which adults, used to the moderation and assuagement of feelings by consciousness and memory, can hardly conceive. Out of this matrix of overwhelming passion the infant's capacity to tolerate its different feelings gradually develops; eventually something like an ego, or a selfhood, is presumed to take shape. But it is a fundamental premise of psychoanalytic thought that these earliest experiences of the psyche – of devastating anger, or hatred, of overwhelming love and gratitude – are never obliterated. They are forgotten, perhaps, but the capacity of the psyche for intense and terrible emotion is kept alive, always capable of being awakened when circumstances confront the person with the sort of experience we describe, for example, as ghastly or horrible.

Now, a fundamental premise of nursing, described by Menzies Lyth (1961), is that it involves dealing with very unpleasant and usually avoided aspects of physical being. As she put it, in part,

> 'Nurses confront suffering and death as few other people do. They work with ill people also under stress... Many nursing tasks are by ordinary standards disgusting, distasteful and frightening. Physical contact with patients may be over-stimulating and disturbing.' (p. 46)

Dealing with the wounded, suppurating and decaying body is the nurse's everyday business. Psychoanalytic thought suggests that this business will arouse and reactivate the nurse's earliest and most powerful emotions. In themselves, these emotions have no names, no context: of their very nature, which belongs to the pre-conceptual era of the psyche, they resist articulation in language. Hence, the tendency both in nursing practice and in nursing research is to overlook or override these aspects to make them 'ordinary' (Parker and Gardner, 1992), to turn the attention towards other concepts, such as 'care', or management techniques, which avoid having to come to terms with the experiences – it is not melodramatic to call them horrific experiences – which the nurse in her everyday practice will encounter. Object-relations psycho-analysis, however, both insists that these experiences are recognised as part of the formed adult self, and offers terminology with which to understand them.

The handover research

Our first project concerned the nursing handover, at that time (Parker and Wiltshire 1995, Parker 1996) under siege as a time-wasting aspect of traditional nursing practice. Here we observed and recorded many handovers in two different hospitals. It became clear that the handover is a complex, multifunctional event, to which many interpretative tools might be brought. Our initial focus was on the way the anecdotes and stories of the nursing shift were reconstituted into a more organised collective narrative (Parker *et al.*, 1992). We then understood this as a group practice of con-tainment made by nurses. Through this process, nurses were enabled to experience their emotions, to have these understood by a group of peers, and to re-experience them, freed of anxiety and fear. This approach brought to light some of the issues that are bound up with the potentially traumatic aspects of nursing practice, and contributed to the greater understanding of nursing experience (Wiltshire and Parker, 1996). In short, the handover had a wide-ranging purpose, including sustaining the mental and emotional equilibrium of the practising nurse.

Menzies Lyth (1961) in the 1950s had examined the various ways the organisation of the traditional hospital attempted to defend the individual nurse from 'anxiety'. These included many institutional arrangements that sought to prevent individual nurses from forming attachments to, or any form of identification with, an individual patient. Times have changed, and different arrangements now prevail in most hospitals. But the need that Menzies Lyth identified – to protect, support or calm the individual nurse who has to deal with emotionally testing material – exists as strongly as ever.

Our assumption was that the handover performed a function which was in excess of its industrial or instrumental role to communicate information to new nurses on the incoming shift. We understood the handover in its guise as a meeting, and we presumed that the ritual aspects of this meeting contributed to the individual nurse's psychological health. We assumed that the importance the handover had for many nurses (we heard nurses claiming how much better they felt after the handover, and how important a good handover was to their well-being), related not just to the discharge of duties, like the handing over of accurate information, but also to the discharge of emotional affects. We felt that the handover was plainly a communal experience that was significant precisely because of its transpersonal elements. Moreover, we felt that the meaning of the handover experience tended to reside in aspects that were never overtly acknowledged.

But how to think about this? If we were to persuade anyone of the value of the traditional handover we would need more than the testimony of the nurses we were collecting, although that testimony clearly counted for a good deal. How would we establish that 'something was going on' in the handover that was as important as the transmission of essential information? Our premise is one we have already indicated: that nursing is for the individual nurse a disturbing experience which has the potential to arouse strong and unmoderated, because archaic, emotions. Drawing partly on the anthropological thought of Mary Douglas (1970), psychoanalysis was able to pinpoint a key aspect of what makes dealing with the sick and injured body disturbing. Douglas suggested that our fundamental act of understanding the world is to put boundaries around things. Moreover, she suggested, the human body is the fundamental metaphor to which we constantly recur. The suppurating, bleeding or wounded body 'embodies' (literally) the transgression or obliteration of boundaries and thus tends to lay siege to the capacity for thought. The psychoanalyst Julia Kristeva (1982), drawing on Douglas, developed the concept of abjection to describe those aspects of experience in which the capacity to relate to something as to an object is put in abeyance. The notion of abjection is now used in nursing and other literature.

However, the fundamental psychoanalytic framework of our understanding came from the work of Wilfred Bion and the useful notion of containing. If an infant has an intolerable anxiety, psychoanalytic theory suggests that he or she deals with it by projecting it into the mother (in ordinary language, the mother is made to feel the emotion the infant is experiencing.) Some mothers – or most mothers on occasion – are unable to deal with this emotion, and reject it, having some such thought, Bion suggests, as an impatient 'I don't know what's the matter with the child'. The effect of the mother rejecting the infant's emotion is to leave the child stranded, weltering in its own feelings. But if the mother is able to experience the child's emotion (Bion speaks of it as 'dread'), moderating it with her own experience and calm, this calm can be communicated to the infant, who thus learns that such feelings are not the be all and end all. In Bion's words,

> 'If the projection is not accepted by the mother the infant feels that its feeling that it is dying is stripped of such meaning as it has. It therefore reintrojects, not a fear of dying made tolerable, but a nameless dread.' (Bion, 1993: 116)

A shorthand term for the capacity to take in and moderate powerfully destructive emotions is 'containing'. Bion elaborated the notion of containing in a variety of contexts, including the social group. His notion, it is important to stress, has nothing in common with the managerial notion of containment as 'damage limitation': indeed it is quite the reverse. We found his a helpful idea to explain the psychological processes that were taking place within the handover meeting. In a successful handover, distressing emotions are conveyed by the individual nurse speakers, and these are accepted by the group. It is not necessary for the group to express overtly any sympathy towards the speaker, or indeed for a speaker to spell out her distress: what matters is the calm and routinised acceptance within the group of the experience. In other words, the function of the group is analogous to the function of the nursing mother. Just as the mother says, implicitly, to the infant, 'what you are feeling may seem terrible to you, but it is really not so terrible to me, and you will get over it', so the nursing group routinises, or, to use our phrase, 'makes ordinary', the experience of the nurse.

Bion defined the turbulent emotions that the infant experiences as 'beta elements' (he chose this mathematical term as a 'working tool' to be free of the encrustations of previous psychoanalytic theory).

He suggested that the process through which such emotions went when accepted by and made ordinary by the mother was what he called alpha function. Through the exercise of 'alpha function', beta elements become alpha elements, and are now able, he suggested, to be 'thought'. Thus he developed what he called 'a theory of thinking'. Since these are merely terms, concepts, metaphors, one might reformulate this idea in a number of guises – one might say, for example, that containment enables the abject to become the object, and mean more or less the same thing. It is in the nature of this research that terms do not refer to fixed, immutable, verifiable entities, but are instead groping attempts to comprehend the mutable, mysterious complexity of experience.

If the mother is not receptive, then without containment the infant, Bion writes, introjects 'nameless dread'. He thus links naming, conceptualisation, words, to the process of alpha functioning. This may in turn throw some light on an important aspect of the handover, for typically the handover is full of stories, or story fragments. In fact its form constitutes an invitation to each nurse to tell the story of each patient under her or his care. These story fragments are often commented on by other nurses, added to, or (sometimes) disputed, until, within the time constraints, a coherent account of a patient's condition or progress is agreed upon or produced. Since this is a mediated and sometimes rather complex process, we thought it plausible to call this a 'collective narrative'.

Narrative and the stoma patient

In our work, then, we have assumed that unconscious and powerful emotions are at work whenever the body and damage to the body is in question. In our second major project, we turned our attention to both patients and nurses who together deal with a particularly traumatic bodily event, the acquisition of a stoma. Here our assumption was that each person takes their body for granted – that it is invisible, in Leder's (1992) well-known phrase. But the surgery that leads to the acquisition of a stoma renders the body, and the functioning of normally invisible bodily processes, literally visible. The processes of digestion and evacuation, normally concealed, become externalised, and require fairly constant psychological attention. This drastic rupture in the ongoing and taken-for-granted aspects of bodily being, it is generally agreed, has profound psychological consequences. Professional help is often required if the change is to be smoothly negotiated, if the patient is to take up normal life again.

In our research we interviewed stomal therapy nurses, and stoma patients in order to understand how, and how successfully, this transition was negotiated. As with the handover study, we have gathered a large amount of empirical evidence, through focus group discussions and interviews with both stoma patients and with stomal therapy nurses. Thinking about this material in psycho-analytic terms has enabled us to interpret the everyday technical management practices of nurses as simultaneously a process of psychological containing. A key concept we have developed is that of 'aphoristic containment': a process whereby verbal acknow-ledgement is given to the abjective or terrible at the same time as it is introduced into the order of the everyday and thinkable (Parker *et al.*, 2000).

In this research the notion of story was useful in a different, broader way. We assumed that everyone tends to tell themselves something that might be called a story of their life. We would affirm that this is a story, not a narrative, precisely because it is fluid, constantly revised and reformulated, depending on circumstances, and rarely put into final form. With the acquisition of a stoma, a person's bodily and psychological life is revolutionised, and a new story about the self and the body needs to be developed. It was our assumption that the kind of story a person tells themselves about their new condition is a vital factor in their therapeutic progress, and may make the difference between permanent psychological wounding, reclusive retreat from society, and effective psychologi-cal and social adjustment. Whether this is so or not, we believe that a coming to terms with the stoma is usually achieved through the creation of a new self-making embodiment story. The caesura that the stoma makes in a life is thus bridged or knitted together by the self's story-making capacity. Thus we turned our attention to the therapeutic efficacy of story-making within the individual psycho-logical life.

This project grew out of an earlier piece of research in which one of us (Parker, 1996) encountered a person whom we called Amelia

Curtis. Originally, Amelia Curtis, like many stoma patients, was disgusted and horrified by her new condition. She felt humiliated and a social outcast. Amelia thought of herself as a straightforward and rather unimaginative person. But she was able to speak about the way that she gained a sense of control over her sense of the sordidness of her condition – and this involved the creative use of the imagination. She dealt with her disgust by imagining the stoma as a baby, by treating the stoma tenderly, and by ritualising her daily cleansing activities. Here again the notion of 'containing' might have been applied, since Amelia, quite unconsciously, was offering to the stoma, a part of herself, the kind of comforting, calming presence that enabled another part of herself to come to terms with her condition. It is interesting that Amelia was a person who thought of herself as putting things in 'boxes', although she had never heard of the concept of containing.

Symbols and metaphors play important parts in our psychological life and are immensely important, we suggest, when bodily disruption causes a person psychological distress. A stoma, which breaks the surface of the body, and through all the accustomed boundaries of the self, raises the most primitive and atavistic of emotions. Excreta on the outside of the body is perhaps the keenest example one could give of 'abjection'. The sense of smell is the most direct, most unmediated of our senses. Because it tends to bypass thought and reflection, it is the sense that is most akin to what Bion defined as the psychological beta elements. For these elements to be contained, to be moderated, to enter into the reconstituted and accepting self, a great deal of psychological work must be done. This conversion of beta elements into alpha elements is done by a variety of means, and the role of the stoma nurse can be critical.

We gathered evidence that much of this work consisted in the patients' spontaneous creation of stories around the stoma. Often this story featured the stoma as its protagonist, and often, too, this protagonist – conceived therefore as an active agent – was named. One interviewee, for example, told us 'I call him Oscar, because he's wild(e)'. A great deal is compressed into that name. Another person said she had named hers Jack, 'because that's the name of the surgeon, and I hate him'. Another constructed a whole story around the stoma as a person, saying that he had introduced his children to it as if it were a new member of the family. This enabled the children to include the noises made by the involuntary excretory activities as part of the conversation of ordinary life. To be able to share jokes about the stoma was an essential part of the accommodation process, for jokes, as Freud himself pointed out, make a great saving of psychological energy, which might otherwise be expended in self-absorption and remorse.

Reflections

In our work, therefore, we have employed a variety of terms and concepts. We have sought here to show how notions of story and narrative can play an important role in nursing research, and also to suggest how these terms need to be thought about and defined with some degree of care. We have tried in our work to marry or amalgamate our view of the importance of story-making activities in the psychological life with psychoanalytic theories which address the vital issue, central to nursing, of how disgusting and stressful work, painful and humiliating conditions, can be dealt with both by the nurse and by the patient.

What we would emphasise, however, is that the psychological terms and concepts we are employing do not in any sense belong to the real or verifiable world. Indeed, they are in themselves metaphors, or stories. One might call them fictive, in the sense that each psychoanalytic writer attempts in his or her own way to codify, and thereby partially to explain, phenomena of human experience. We do not use our research material therefore as documentation to substantiate, say, Bion's theory of containment, as one might use the research generated in a laboratory to substantiate a biochemical proposition. Bion, like all psychoanalytic thinkers, emphasises that his names are merely tools with which to come to terms with experience. Thus we find it permissible, in this kind of research, to draw concepts from different psychoanalytic perspectives, and to ignore differences in orientation, when we feel that the terms and concepts provide useful ways of understanding our material.

'Understanding' is a word that needs to be stressed. The goal of nursing research as we practise it is not to produce results that can be acted upon (though this may be a gratifying outcome of some research). It is to produce ideas and concepts that enable nurses and fellow nurse researchers to think more deeply about their practices – and, we might add, about the body, about embodiment, and about patienthood. Much of the material we have gathered is deeply affecting. It testifies to human suffering, to human kindness and inventiveness. The nursing researcher will often be a privileged witness and custodian of such material. The task is to find ways in which this – for which we have proposed the term, the metaphor, of story – can be turned into something that is understood, that can be thought – into narrative. In this sense, qualitative research seeks to destabilise and disturb taken-for-granted practices and assumptions, to give another shake to the kaleidoscope of experience.

References

Atkinson, P. & Silverman, D. (1997) Kundera's immortality: The interview society and the invention of the self. *Qualitative Inquiry* **3** (3): 304–25.

Benner, P. (1991) The role of experience, narrative, and community in skilled ethical comportment. *Advances in Nursing Science* **14** (2): 1–21.

Bion, W.R. (1961) *Experiences in Groups and Other Papers*. London: Tavistock.

Bion, W.R. (1993) *A Theory of Thinking. Second Thoughts: Selected Papers on Psycho-analysis*. Northvale, New Jersey.

Bowles, N. (1995) Story telling: a search for meaning within nursing practice. *Nurse Education Today* **15** (5): 365–9.

Canales, M. (1997) Narrative interaction: creating a space for therapeutic communication. *Issues in Mental Health Nursing* **18** (5): 477–94.

Clark, M.C. & Standard, P.L. (1997) The caregiving story: how the narrative approach informs caregiving burden. *Issues in Mental Health Nursing* **18** (2): 87–97.

Crowe, M. (1998) The power of the word: some post-structural considerations of qualitative approaches in nursing research. *Journal of Advanced Nursing* **28** (2): 339–44.

Darbyshire, P. (1994) Reality bites: the theory and practice of nursing narratives. *Nursing Times* **90** (4): 31–3.

Douglas, M. (1970) *Purity and Danger: An Analysis of Concepts of Pollution and Taboo*. Harmondsworth: Penguin.

Facione, N.C. & Giancarlo, C.A. (1998) Narratives of breast symptom discovery and cancer diagnosis: psychologic risk for advanced cancer at diagnosis. *Cancer Nursing* **231** (6): 430–40.

Frank, A. (1995) *The Wounded Storyteller: Body, Illness, and Ethics*. Chicago: University of Chicago Press.

Freud, S. (1912) *The Dynamics of Transference*, Standard Edition of the Works of Sigmund Freud, Vol. 12, pp. 97–108.

Gadow, S. (1995) Narrative and exploration: toward a poetics of knowledge in nursing. *Nursing Inquiry* **2** (4): 211–14.

Gadow, S. (1999) Relational narrative: the postmodern turn in nursing ethics. *Scholarly Inquiry for Nursing Practice* **13** (1): 57–70.

Harden, J. (2000) Language, discourse and the chronotope: applying literary theory to the narratives in health care. *Journal of Advanced Nursing* **31** (3): 506–12.

Hunter, K.M. (1991) *Doctors' Stories: The Narrative Structure of Medical Knowledge*. Princeton, NJ: Princeton University Press.

Klein, M. (1935) A contribution to the psychogenesis of manic–depressive states. *The Writings of Melanie Klein*, Vol. 1, pp. 262–89.

Kleinman, A. (1988) *The Illness Narratives, Suffering, Healing and the Human Condition*. New York: Basic Books.

Kristeva, J. (1982) *Powers of Horror* (Leon Roudiez, trans.). New York: Columbia University Press.

Leder, D. (1992) A tale of two bodies: the cartesian corpse and the lived body. In D. Leder (ed.) *The Body in Medical Thought and Practice*. Dordrecht: Kluwer Academic, pp. 17–36.

McLeod, A.A. (1997) Resisting invitations to depression: a narrative approach to family nursing. *Journal of Family Nursing* **3** (4): 397–406.

Menzies Lyth I. (1961) Nurses under stress. *Nursing Times* **3** (February). Reprinted in *Containing Anxiety in Institutions. Selected Essays*, Vol. 1. London: Free Association Books, 1988, pp. 100–104.

Moules, N.J. & Amundson, J.K. (1997) Grief – an invitation to inertia: a narrative approach to working with grief. *Journal of Family Nursing* **3** (4): 378–93.

Nehls, N. (1995) Narrative pedagogy: rethinking nursing education. *Journal of Nursing Education* **34** (5): 204–10.

Parker, J. (1996) Bodily concealment and the visible stoma. *Hysteric*, 1996, 2: 9–16.

Parker, J. & Gardner, G. (1992) The silence and the silencing of the nurse's voice: a reading of patient progress notes. *The Australian Journal of Advanced Nursing* **9** (2): 3–9.

Parker, J. & Wiltshire, J. (1995) The handover: three models of nursing practice knowledge. In G. Gray & R. Pratt (eds) *Scholarship in the Discipline of Nursing*. Melbourne: Churchill Livingstone, pp. 151–68.

Parker, J. (1996) Handovers in a changing health climate. *Australian Nursing Journal* **4** (5): 22–6.

Parker, J., Gardner, G. & Wiltshire, J. (1992) Handover: the collective narrative of nursing practice. *The Australian Journal of Advanced Nursing* **9** (3): 31–7.

Parker, J., Wright, R. & Peerson, A. (2000) The changing health care environment and the visibility of stomal therapy nursing. *Journal of Stomal Therapy Australia* **20** (3): 21–3.

Sakalys, J.A. (2000) The political role of illness narratives. *Journal of Advanced Nursing* **31** (6): 1469–75.

Sandelowski, M. (1991) Telling stories: narrative approaches in qualitative research. *IMAGE: Journal of Nursing Scholarship* **23**: 161–6.

Sandelowski, M. (1994) We are the stories we tell: narrative knowing in nursing practice. *Journal of Holistic Nursing* **12** (1) 23–33.

Stevens, P.E. (1996) Struggles with symptoms: women's narratives of managing HIV illness. *Journal of Holistic Nursing* **14** (2): 142–60.

Svedlund, M., Danielson, E. & Norberg, A. (1999) Nurses' narrations about caring for inpatients with acute myocardial infarction. *Intensive and Critical Care Nursing* **15** (1): 34–43.

Tanner, C.A., Benner, P., Chesla, C. & Gordon, D.R. (1993) The phenomenology of knowing the patient. *IMAGE: Journal of Nursing Scholarship* **25** (4): 273–80.

Wiltshire, J. & Parker, J. (1996) Containing abjection in nursing: the end of shift handover as a site of containment. *Nursing Inquiry* **3**: 23–9.

Wiltshire, J. (1995) Telling a story, writing a narrative: terminology in health care. *Nursing Inquiry* **2**: 75–85.

CHAPTER 7

Rational solutions and unreliable narrators: content, structure and voice in narrative research

Lioness Ayres & Suzanne Poirier

Narrative research is an omnibus term that refers to a variety of approaches to analysis. Some authors describe narrative research as 'any study that uses or analyzes narrative materials' (Lieblich *et al.*, 1998: 2), a definition so broad that it stretches from content analysis to life history research. Others define narrative research as the practice of 'thinking about data as stories' (Coffey & Atkinson, 1996: 56). Researchers who think about their data as stories may choose amongst a variety of analytic strategies designed to interpret the form (structure) or function (purpose) of stories (Mishler, 1986). For this chapter, narrative research is defined by process: the data are conceived as stories, and narrative methods are used to explore not only 'what was said in [the] data but how it was said' (Coffey & Atkinson, 1996: 83).

The underlying assumption of narrative methods is that interpretation extends beyond what Poirier and Ayres call 'the tale' (1997: 552); the way in which the tale is told conveys additional meaning. Story-tellers select, order and report events in ways that explain their situations or circumstances. By attending to the way the tale is told, narrative researchers are able to explore meanings implicit in the telling. One strategy for such exploration is over-reading (Kermode, 1981; Poirier & Ayres, 1997); that is, reading that searches for meanings both explicit and implicit. Stories are built of many familiar narrative elements such as plot, character, setting and point of view (Ayres & Poirier, 1996; Poirier & Ayres, 1997). This chapter explores the role of three of those elements – content, structure and voice – in narrative research. Content refers to choices about what to tell and what to withhold; structural choices include where a story begins and how it ends; the use of voice establishes the narrator's authority or expertise. The way researchers as readers respond to content, structure and voice plays a crucial role in the trustworthiness of the resulting interpretation.

The purpose of this chapter is to provide some examples of content, structure and voice in narratives of family caregivers, and to illustrate the way these three elements influenced one researcher's interpretation of those narratives. In the study of family caregiving described below, the use of a narrative approach sheds new light on caregivers' experience and helped to explain why caregivers in externally similar circumstances described very different meanings for and affective responses to caregiving (Ayres, 2000a, b). Since nurses are often engaged in understanding and treating human responses to health and illness, and since those responses are often highly variable across externally similar circumstances, an understanding of narrative is useful both for nurses and for clinicians. In addition, because nurses, like family caregivers, are persons who make meaning out of their experiences in caring for others, narrative provides a useful avenue to understand and communicate nursing knowledge (see also Boykin & Schoenhofer, 1991).

Rationality and secrets

No story is a perfect mirror of experience. Although literary narrators may feign or claim omniscience about their creations, readers who receive experience at second hand must perforce be satisfied with such information as the narrator provides. For this reason, all stories contain secrets. According to Kermode (1981: 84), secrets are aspects of the text that are not 'rationally soluble', that is, even in the simplest story, some aspects of the narrative cannot be known from the evidence in the text. For example, in the story of Little Red Ridinghood, readers never know whether Red Ridinghood had other siblings who could have accompanied her to her grandmother's house; neither does the reader learn why this frail old woman lives in an isolated cottage in a dangerous wood rather than with her extended family. In addition, secrets are virtual, that is, they do not exist in the text as such but arise out of the interaction of the tale and the manner of its telling with the intellect of the reader or researcher (Iser, 1980; Bruner, 1986; Ayres & Poirier, 1996). In the story of Little Red Ridinghood, a family researcher would see different secrets from those that a rural sociologist would see. Thus secrets are dependent on, and arise from, both the story and the mind of the interpreter.

Certain narrative strategies point to the presence of a secret. One narrator may say the same thing many times, as with Lady Gertrude's criticism in *Hamlet* that '[t]he lady doth protest too much'. Another narrator may choose to omit parts of a story that the reader or researcher would expect to be told (Poirier & Ayres, 1997). The full meaning of these stories can be missed if the reader attends only to the words and not to the story as a whole.

For qualitative researchers, additional loss of meaning may occur in analytic strategies that rely only on words that have been decontextualized from their original source. These decontextualized segments, compared only with one another and not returned to their original context, may oversimplify informants' stories (see, for example, Kavanaugh & Ayres, 1998). Oversimplified interpretations are untrustworthy. They exclude relevant dimensions of meaning from the interpretation, and are a particular risk when data reduction strategies are used for thematic analysis. For this reason, it is crucial for qualitative researchers who use data coding and categorization strategies to identify and use strategies that address the narrative as it was produced, as a coherent whole. The remainder of this chapter describes issues that arose in a study of family caregiving that combined narrative and coding strategies.

Content and inconsistency[1]

In my qualitative study of family caregiving, I used two complementary strategies: data coding and reduction, and narrative analysis. Details of the integration of these two analytic strategies have been described elsewhere (Ayres, 2000a, b). Data coding and reduction were used to identify a range of themes that occurred across cases and to describe the range of variation among caregivers' responses across those themes. Narrative analysis was used to describe the ways those themes combined into patterns characteristic of individual caregivers' experiences. My plan was to develop a scheme of mutually exclusive themes and sub-themes for family caregiving, to name those themes and sub-themes, and to compare the patterns those subthemes created across caregivers' accounts by using matrices as described by Miles and Huberman (1994). I intended to integrate this matrix display, similar to the one described by Knafl and Ayres (1996) for use with a family data set, with blocks of text from the interviews, and with memos that described the important 'secrets', which were defined for this study as repetitions, evasions, omissions and incongruencies in individual accounts.

One important theme in all of the interviews was the caregiver's view of the care receiver's moral accountability. On this theme, I identified three views: ordinary, absolved and blameworthy. Ordinary care receivers were held to the same standards that caregivers used for other family members. Absolved care receivers were excused from many troubling or disturbing behaviors on the basis of sick role permissions; caregivers forgave them because their actions were seen as involuntary symptoms or consequences of illness. Caregivers often used the words 'it's not his fault' or 'she can't help it' to qualify descriptions of absolved care receivers' words or actions. In contrast, blameworthy care receivers were described as deliberately choosing to thwart or undermine the caregiver's work or well-being. The assumption underlying this thematic analysis was that the three themes of ordinary, absolved and blameworthy care receivers were mutually exclusive. Rationally, a care receiver could not be both responsible and not responsible for his or her actions. In the stories told by some caregivers, however, this rational expectation was not fulfilled. Some caregivers defined the care receiver as accountable in some parts of the interview, absolved in others, and blameworthy in yet others, often in the context of the same or similar actions. For example, one woman, Ms G, described her husband after brain surgery:

'They operated on him first thing in the morning and he was in the hospital about a week, a little over a week. Was absolutely miserable, was horrible to everybody in the hospital. Including me. He was very, very cruel to me. Very paranoid, after the surgery. Accused me of all sorts of things. It was very hard for me. And I finally remember going to the nurses and saying, you know, "I need someone to tell me, is this just temporary or is this the way he's gonna be now?" And they said, "Nonono, this is temporary, because of the medication," And he's got the tube – and he had the tube in his head for drainage and everything – and he pretty much stayed [horrible] for quite a while, probably about a month, month and a half. Until I finally told him, "I can't do this anymore." I told him, "I didn't do this to you. I'm sorry if you thought I was gonna die first. I thought I was gonna die first, too. But that's not the way it worked out, but I didn't do this to you, and you're not gonna take it out on me." '

As this example demonstrates, Ms G initially interpreted her husband's behavior as the result of treatment or medication. Her strategy to manage the behavior, to explain to him why he should not 'take it out' on her, is inappropriate to such an explanation, and suggests that she has responded to his behavior as she would to a person whose cognitive functions were intact. Instead, she held him to the same standards as persons who had not had brain surgery. Based on these two conflicting explanations for his cruelty and paranoia, Ms G often had inconsistent expectations for her husband's behavior, and these unmet expectations in turn often left her hurt and angry.

Ms G alluded throughout the interview to the unhappiness and confusion these two views of her husband's behavior caused:

'Or he, because he doesn't remember things well, he'll remember something that I did but he remembers it differently than it was. And so you try to explain to him that that's not how it happened and then he gets angry at me. He said there was a long period of time – weeks – a month – where I never asked him how he was. Now I know that's not true. But in HIS mind I hadn't asked him, and so of course he told his therapist this. So then he proceeds to tell me, "Well, MY therapist told me why you are the way you are." And of course see that makes the hairs on the back of my neck sit up because I think to myself, "I didn't do anything wrong." You know, maybe you just didn't remember it. But then if I say that, then he gets angry with me, 'cause I'm saying that he doesn't remember things correctly – when he doesn't . . . And it angered me. And it still does.'

In the previous extract, Ms G interprets her husband's actions as though he were both absolved (problem behavior due to medication) and ordinary (problem behavior due to underlying resentment or jealousy). In this example, Ms G recognizes that her husband's ability to interpret events, in this case his inability to remember a caring behavior of hers, is a consequence of brain damage. In my original reductionist scheme, I would have interpreted this explanation as absolution of Mr G. However, because Mr G disagrees with Ms G's interpretation of events (that he has misremembered what she did because of his disability), Ms G withholds absolution and holds him accountable for his inability to remember that he cannot remember. That is, because Mr G does not see himself as needing absolution, a failure of insight also consequent to Mr G's disability, Ms G holds him to the same standard of behaviour as she would any other person. By this standard, her husband has been unjust to her and the injustice is exacerbated when he communicates his version of reality to his therapist. In the face of similar incidents, Ms G began to wonder if in fact her husband was deliberately causing her pain and that, as a moral agent, he was blameworthy.

Taken as a whole, the interview provided some evidence that Ms G held her husband blameworthy, some evidence that she absolved him, and some evidence that she saw him as normal or ordinary. The simplest solution would have been to describe Ms G's view of her husband as absolved since her most direct statements tended to excuse him. For example, she said 'I lost him as soon as [the surgeon] opened up that head of his.' Any single resolution would have foreclosed a full understanding of Ms G and her struggles to make sense of her husband's actions and resulted in an inadequate interpretation.

Sandelowski (1993) inveighed against using a reliability standard in qualitative research. In particular, Sandelowski has challenged researchers to reconsider inconsistency within informants' accounts as evidence against validity or trustworthiness. Discussing discrepant versions of the same life event, Sandelowski recommended that the researcher, rather than 'dismiss[ing] the storyteller as an unreliable informant ... consider whether the versions are truly inconsistent ... or if inconsistent, why discrepancies exist, or whether the ... discrepant accounts even represent the same story' (p. 4). In Ms G's story, her inconsistency points to a secret in her story.

Ms G describes one rational solution to her problem, saying, '... How much of this is really him, I don't know. I have no way of knowing.' Yet her strategies to manage his behaviors, particularly her reliance on psychotherapy, reasoned discourse and inter-personal negotiation, imply a belief that her husband is able to understand information and respond to it as a normal and ordinary person. Logically, then, if her husband is able to understand and respond, and to control his behavior, the injustice of his actions and the suffering they cause Ms G must be deliberately chosen.

Ms G's beliefs about her husband's moral accountability are discrepant. Overreading of her comments in the contexts from which they were taken (a strategy that might not be used in all kinds of thematic analysis) showed patterns in her inconsistency. When she thought about Mr G in the context of his illness, she absolved him; when she thought about him in the context of his behavior towards her, she blamed him for his injustice. Ms G has at least two competing, contradictory stories about her husband's moral accountability. I was able to explain this inconsistency in Ms G's story, although not to resolve it, because every statement Ms G made about her husband's accountability was examined, and because each statement was interpreted in the context of the rest of the interview. In this process, I looked not only for statements of explanation or intent, but also for evidence of those ideas expressed in actions.

I learned a great deal from Ms G's interview, not only about secrets and rational solutions, but also about the influence of meaning on caregivers' affective responses. Ms G struggled con-stantly to make sense of her husband's behavior towards her, responding sometimes with anger, sometimes with guilt, sometimes with bewilderment. Her lack of a coherent explanation for his actions interfered with her ability to manage her own affective responses and safeguard her psychological well-being while pro-viding care for her husband. I found that caregivers made choices about the structure of their stories in order to manage their affective responses to caregiving. Structural choices were especially evident when I asked caregivers about the future, especially about a future in which the care receiver's health deteriorated.

Structure and imposed plots

I came to this study of family caregiving from a clinical practice in home health and hospice nursing, which influenced my expectations for caregivers' stories. In particular, my clinical experience convinced me that coordinated care between home health, hospital and hospice led to the best outcomes for patients and their families, and that coordination among providers worked best when clients and families participated together in planning for the inevitable deterioration of the care receiver's condition. I also believed that, in order for clients' and families' treatment wishes to be effective, those wishes needed to be both explicit and documented well in advance of need. Based on these beliefs, I came to this study with strong opinions about the desirability not only of written advance directives but also of contingency plans for caregivers in the event that the condition of the care receiver changed suddenly.

Brooks (1984) has suggested, with homage to Freud, that the resolution of tension in all stories is quiescence, and the prototype of such quiescence is death. Certainly, death was the likely end for most stories of family caregiving. For the caregivers I interviewed, all of whom were caring for family members with chronic or terminal illnesses, the caregiving story could only end in two ways: with the death of the caregiver or the death of the care receiver. Even caregivers who planned to institutionalize the care receiver understood that institutionalization did not end the caregiving story, but only changed its venue. For the caregivers in my study, therefore, thinking about the future meant thinking explicitly about their own deaths or anticipating the deterioration and death of a person dearly loved, and who would be sorely missed. Many caregivers found such speculations morbid and resisted them. They described these thoughts as 'dwelling', an activity they found incompatible with psychological well-being. Surrender to dwelling, caregivers stated unequivocally, led to unacceptable affective responses such as despair or paralyzing sadness.

A few caregivers, when asked about the future, described in clear and rational language their plans for life after caregiving. Others, especially parents of teenagers with disabilities, answered questions about the future with details of estate planning or guardianship. But some informants, although they appeared to be in good health and to have a reasonable expectation to survive the care receiver by many years, said that they themselves expected to die first. This choice of ending was inconsistent with caregiving stories from my clinical experience. Nevertheless, caregivers like Tony Brown (Poirier & Ayres, 1997: 553), who had every reason to expect to outlive his severely disabled wife, said of the future, 'I think she's gonna bury me.'

Other caregivers, including a middle-aged woman caring for her mother, refused to speculate, saying, 'You know, I could die – you know, even though she in that shape [bedridden, tube-fed, with heart and kidney disease], I still could die before she did . . . You're not sure [of] tomorrow – you ain't even sure [of] this afternoon.' A woman caring for her husband repudiated both dwelling and the virtues of advance directives:

> 'You know, I don't know that you dwell on the long term part of it. It's the one day at a time part. It's One! Day! At a time! If you begin to sit and think and worry about what's – you don't *know* what's going to happen. You can make all the preparations in the world, what's gonna happen's gonna happen.'

These stories did not make sense to me. I thought they, and their narrators, were irrational. I doubted that these healthy caregivers would die before their often seriously ill care receivers, and I doubted also that they actually expected to do so.

That impression, accurate though it might have been, missed the point. These caregivers were characters in the midst of stories, and those stories were driven by both external circumstances and their own, internal logic. According to Culler (1981: 178), narrative operates according to a 'double logic' so that at times a story's 'events are justified by their appropriateness to a narrative structure'. In these stories, whose endings I initially dismissed as irrational, Culler's double logic operated to allow caregivers to look away from a more rational but painful conclusion. When I asked caregivers for their stories, those stories unfolded in the context of the narrator's identity as caregiver. Thus, by the logic of the plot, the end of caregiving meant the end of the story, and, by extension, the end of the narrator. When I pressured caregivers to predict the end of their stories, they described endings that resolved the narrative difficulty and avoided the unacceptable dwelling on bad outcomes by anticipating their own quiescence instead.

But this is the logic of plot, not the logic of real life. When I asked caregivers about the future apart from caregiving, they described activities that implied their own persistence in time. They bought insurance, they hoped for grandchildren, they planted gardens and fixed the roof. The inconsistency in their narratives came from my questions, in which the deterioration and death of the care receiver were made explicit. The ends of individual caregivers' stories, by contrast, were unknown and secret. Neither did their narrators choose to dwell on the end of the story or the stories that might come after. Some caregivers were quite aware of their narrative choices and the reasons for them. One said, 'I can't imagine what my life will be like without [the care receiver], so I don't.' Another woman, clearly put out by my apparent inability to recognize the necessities of her story, said, 'I try not to [think about it].'

The explanatory power of narrative is retroactive; that is, events in stories take on significance based on the story's end (Brooks, 1984; Polkinghorne, 1988). My ideas about advance directives and future planning came from stories that were over, and often had ended in the death of the care receiver. Many had ended badly, with extraordinary means used to preserve life at the cost of terrible suffering or financial hardship; with undignified, lonely deaths in hospital emergency rooms or intensive care units; with rib fractures, burns, and bruises; and with caregivers who said, 'If only I had known.' Those endings gave explanatory power to my story and provided the logic for its plot. But this was my story, different from the stories told by the caregivers in my research. Absent the explanatory function of the actual end of their stories, caregivers either substituted their own deaths or left their stories open-ended.

By trying to impose my story on theirs, I had attempted to make their stories suit the logic of my own plot. Once I recognized that my informants and I were working from different plots, and that my ideas of endings interfered with informants' sense of their own stories, the barriers to a rational solution were overcome. Although this explanation did not lead to strategies to persuade caregivers to do more advance planning, I was able to understand caregivers' resistance to advance planning as an outgrowth of the meaning of caregiving as well as an important strategy for maintaining a positive affect. Thus advance planning, which I privileged from my clinical perspective, had a lower priority for caregivers, for whom 'dwelling' on possible futures interfered with their ability to manage and often appreciate the present.

Narrative voice and unreliable narrators

The unreliable narrator is a literary device, and the term casts no aspersions on the 'integrity of the informant' (Lincoln & Guba, 1985: 315). Booth (1983: 158) said of the fictional narrator that 'the total effect' of the tale is transformed by the reader's evaluation of the 'moral and intellectual qualities of the narrator'. Regarding the narrators' intellectual qualities, Booth considered unreliable those narrators who are mistaken, misinformed, or unable to understand the circumstances or events of the story. Examples of unreliable narrators in literature include Salinger's Holden Caulfield (the naive youth of *Catcher in the Rye*, J.D. Salinger) or Faulkner's Benjy (the mentally retarded adult in, *The Sound and the Fury*, William Faulkner). An unreliable narrator who is neither mistaken nor misinformed may yet lack information necessary to understand the story of which he or she is a part. In this regard, many interview informants can be seen as unreliable, first and most obviously with regard to the analysis as a whole (see, for example, Sandelowski, 1993; Ayres & Poirier, 1996). In addition, participants in nursing research may understand health and illness very differently from the researcher.

The reader's evaluation of a narrator's 'moral qualities' also influences the interpretation of a story. Some fictional narratives created using the voice of characters 'whose conduct the author deeply deplores ... [and who are presented] through the seductive medium of their own self-defending rhetoric' (Booth, 1983: 388–9). One example of a deplorable narrator is Nabokov's *tour de force* creation of Humbert Humbert in *Lolita*. Nabokov uses Humbert's voice in the first person to stunning effect, allowing Humbert's self-defending rhetoric to damn him in the reader's eye. Humbert, who writes of himself as an injured innocent, putty in the hands of the demon nymphet Lolita, reveals himself as an opportunist and pedophile who marries a woman he despises in the hope of seducing her 12-year-old daughter. *Lolita* is the story of Humbert and Lolita, beginning with their first meeting and ending in Humbert's death. Although internally consistent on its own terms, Humbert's account flies in the face of the reader's moral values. In his own eyes, Humbert is blameless, innocent, even oppressed. To the reader, outraged at Humbert's justifications for unconscionable acts, attributions of innocence and culpability, oppressed and oppressor, protagonist and antagonist are reversed.

None of the participants in my research were deplorable as the reader deplores Humbert, but some caregivers' stories shared narrative attributes with his. That is, some of the stories told by family caregivers used self-defending rhetoric to describe behaviors that met Phillips *et al.*'s (1995) criteria for poor quality care. These informants described care that, although it 'could not be classified legally as abuse or neglect [was] nonetheless ... sporadic, insensitive, [or] inattentive' (Phillips *et al.*, 1995: 205–206). When caregivers used narrative devices to justify or defend insensitive or inattentive care, I found myself reacting to the 'moral qualities' in these narratives in ways that influenced my interpretations.

Stories of insensitive or inattentive care were told by caregivers who found themselves increasingly unable or unwilling to continue providing care and, in two instances, by caregivers who had already begun preparations for the institutionalization of the care receiver. In all of these stories, events were selected and described to show the care receivers as working against their own best interests as well as the best interests of the caregiver. Care receivers were portrayed as uncooperative, disagreeable, unmanageable and complicit in their own disability. Difficult behaviors were always seen as deliberate efforts to thwart, evade or devalue the caregiver. In these stories, care receivers were all seen as blameworthy and undeserving of good quality care. The authority inherent in the first-person voice served to distract the listener or reader from the missing voice of the care receiver, who was effectively silenced by this narrative strategy. The example below comes from the story of Mr and Ms R. and comes from an interview with Mr R.

Ms R was never sick until her injury a year before. She was active, employed full time in a nursing home, going out with her husband on her days off to shopping malls or restaurants. Mr R describes their life nostalgically, saying, 'We were living it up, for poor people.' Then she began to have back problems. She entered the hospital for diagnostic tests. Somehow, although Mr R offers no details, 'she walked in ... but she came out in an ambulance', paralyzed from the waist down. After some weeks in acute care, Ms R spent three months in a rehabilitation hospital and then came home. She almost immediately developed problems about which Mr R is vague but which seem to have included pressure sores. Ms R returned to the hospital, where she moved back and forth between acute and extended care units for six more months. At the time of the interview she had been home for less than eight weeks.

Ms R's precarious health and severe disability are not the only challenges for Mr R, who has health problems of his own. He has a potentially lethal chronic illness and must spend three mornings a week receiving treatments that include intravenous medication and blood products. His physical care and his medical management are demanding and he must adhere strictly to diet and activity restrictions. He ascribes his ability to thrive despite diagnoses that many would find incapacitating, to his positive attitude. He says that whenever the doctors or nurses ask him how he's doing, he replies, 'I'm fine and dandy!'

Mr R believes in the value of a positive presentation of self – about being fine and dandy– and he has equally strong convictions about other kinds of self-presentations:

'... if you don't show any interest or no motivation, nobody else is either, and you're going to wind up, which is what I want to tell her, "You're just gonna be thrown in a corner! You're gonna be forgotten!"'

There is no evidence that Mr R has ever been 'thrown in a corner', presumably thanks to his own interest and motivation. Similarly, he has nothing but praise for the people who provide care for himself and his wife – his wife has so far not been thrown in the corner, either. Mr R is not operating out of a double standard when he criticizes his wife. He, himself, had major surgery just two weeks before the interview. Although he has resumed most of his presurgery activities, he is dissatisfied with his progress. 'My mind says I'm fine and dandy, but my body doesn't,' he observes. 'I'm dandy mentally ... and I'm trying to make the dandy mentally transfer into the physically.' His motivation is undimmed, but his body so far has failed to keep up.

Mr R bases his ideas about how sick people should think and act on his own success, and when he describes his wife's experience, he identifies her refusal to, as he says, 'make the best of a bad situation', as the root of her failure to improve:

> '...the physical [therapist] thinks ... the thing is to get her upper body strength and he's trying to impress upon her that "You've got to do this," but see there's other factors. She doesn't have the motivation, she doesn't eat, she doesn't – she doesn't have the right attitude, she doesn't... Let me put it like this, it's – my greatest attempt would be to try to make the best of a bad situation. OK. And the harder I try, the worse it gets ... It wound up taking a toll on me that I – I – I wasn't resting properly, I wasn't – I wasn't doing anything properly but for want of a better word sacrificing myself to try to placate her [but] placation didn't work ... It is frustrating and plus the fact that it comes out to a certain amount of *resentment*, and sometimes so much resentment that I have to speak back to her harshly, for example like before you came, she slumped in the bed. But basically I'm not supposed to do anything because [of my activity restrictions], well, OK, it's not too bad, so, let the bed down and the minute you let it down, she has pain. She can't stand to be touched! See, and it's not only that but when the health care people come, they can do it and she'll holler or this that and the other but she won't say nothing. But when I was trying to do it, I had a whole lot of *criticism*. And I was only doing what I was TAUGHT to do! The same things that they were doing! So it just eliminated me doing this, so it – we're to the case where now we are looking for a nursing home, see, because it's just – it – it – it – basically, it's just too much.

Of course, there is more to the story. Not only does Ms R reject the recommendation that she make the best of her situation, not only does she direct criticism and resentment at her husband, not only does she holler and resist Mr R's efforts to make her eat and exercise – to make matters worse she attacks Mr R at the heart of his self-image:

> '… she thinks I'm a phony, because I – I – I'm get up and go, you know, all the time, nothing uncommon for me to get up at 4 o'clock in the morning to go to work, be at work at 5 o'clock, 3 o'clock in the morning, all this sort of thing. And I've always been that way, like I say to her, even in my condition right now, I used to say, prior to [my surgery], "I'm fine and dandy."
>
> "I don't know why you would say that. You're not fine and dandy."
>
> I say, "Of course I am! Because I'm [getting medical treatment], that doesn't mean I'm not fine and dandy!" '

Mr R's care strategies fulfill his warning to people who don't 'show any interest or motivation'. He avoids his wife as much as possible. Her companions are hired caregivers: home health aides and homemakers.

> 'I stay out of it altogether so when [her sitter] comes in the evening, I just go in my room and watch a basketball game or go downstairs and just stay out of the way … because my contact with her in a lot of instances is a lot of resentment … If something is wrong, I'm at fault. I am the guilty party.'

I ask why, with all of his health problems, Mr R had chosen to bring his wife home, but he implies that the choice was not entirely his. He says, 'The point is in a lot of instances I yield to her because I just don't feel like arguing. I'll go like Chamberlain, peace at any price.' Mr R has, like Chamberlain, discovered that he cannot live with the peace agreement he had reached. He will move his wife to a nursing home as soon as a bed becomes available despite her stated opposition to nursing home placement:

> 'She worked in a nursing home, so she was aware of some of the factors that could go on in a nursing home, so she was very adamant about coming home rather than to go into a nursing home.'

He never discloses whether his wife is aware of his current plans to put her into a nursing home – the 'we' in 'we are looking for a nursing home' refers to his home health nurse. Nor does he speculate whether his plan to institutionalize his wife has anything to do with her resentment and criticism.

As a nurse I recognized, but did not support, the portraits of Mr and Ms R to which Mr R's narrative voice directed me. This voice is woven so completely into the events of the tale that its moralizing is seldom heard clearly. Stepping back and reading the text of the interview, I was better able to see that Mr R chose language, interpretations and events that implicated his wife as the author of her own distress. If only she would do something about her attitude, cheer up, be fine and dandy, and give Mr R and his advice the respect they deserve, he would willingly care for her despite his own poor health. Under his direction, Ms R would thrive and improve, as is demonstrated by Mr R's own experience. But if Ms R persists in the error of her ways, Mr R will exile her to a nursing home, in effect throwing her into a corner. Mr R will send his wife to the place she most wishes not to go: the nursing home, which for Ms R is not an abstract terror but a real one, known through first-hand experience. Mr R's narrative suggests that he has done the best he could. Ms R's fate is her own fault and no one else's, a direct consequence of her refusal to see or to be fine and dandy.

A naive reader might respond to the seductiveness of Mr R's story and risk wholesale acceptance of its implicit values, 'yield[ing] to a comfortable identification' with this unreliable narrator (Booth, 1983: 391). The more clinically or narratively sophisticated reader might offer an interpretation of Ms R's behavior that contradicts her husband's. Such an interpretation would re-evaluate Ms R's behavior – the pain, rage, withdrawal, the crying and lost appetite – as symptoms of depression and thus reasonable, familiar and potentially treatable responses to spinal cord injury. There is no evidence in Mr R's account that he has ever considered his wife's behavior to be anything other than evidence of her flawed character. He never mentions whether he had ever made or been offered any other explanations – one of the many secrets in this interview. When asked directly, Mr R rejects the possibility that his poor health might have any influence on his ability to care for his wife. His decision for nursing home placement is never attributed to his incapacity, which is substantial. All of his explanations return to the theme of his wife's refusal to work towards recovery. If Ms R's lack of motivation were attributed to depression, a very different reading of this story would result. The reader might see Ms R as absolved from her behaviors and consequently might question Mr R's justifications for 'speak[ing] back harshly' to his wife, for retreating to his room and leaving her alone, for sending her to the nursing home. In this interpretation, not Ms R but Mr R would be morally suspect.

Conclusion

Narrative secrets are a source of tension for readers and listeners and therefore present a challenge to interpreters. Nurse clinicians and researchers, who in the course of their work hear and interpret many stories, may be tempted to impose rational solutions on secrets and distort the meaning of the original account. The purpose of a narrative approach is to reveal, not resolve, those secrets although resolution sometimes results. In the first example presented here, the rational solution to Ms G's apparent inconsistency uncovered a flaw in the original interpretation; that is, caregivers can and do, albeit at some cost, hold simultaneous yet mutually exclusive views of the care receiver as a moral agent. The difficulty in the interpretation of Ms G's narrative was less unreliability of the narrative than of the reading, a problem caused by the imposition of formal logic on the human heart.

Similarly, caregivers' apparently irrational ideas about the future resulted from inaccurate and unarticulated assumptions in the research design. Once those assumptions were exposed, caregivers' ideas about the future no longer seemed unreasonable. In the two examples, Ms G's views of her husband as a moral agent and caregivers' ideas about the future, interpretative difficulties that initially seemed inherent in the narrative were instead products of the interpretation. Neither Ms G nor the research participants whose ideas about the future I questioned were in fact unreliable; rather, it was my interpretation that was flawed. The reliability of Mr R's narrative, in contrast, is more open to question.

Researchers bring broader or more theoretical perspectives to informants' accounts (Sandelowski, 1993). Such an understanding is a desirable outcome of qualitative research. It is less common, and more controversial, for researchers to offer an interpretation that competes with the explanation offered by an informant; that is, it is uncommon for qualitative researchers to openly question a narrator's reliability. Nurses and qualitative researchers are disposed to view informants as the ultimate experts on their own experience. When evidence in the text leads the researcher to very different conclusions from those expressed by the informant, those conclusions must be supported by strong evidence within the text as well as by the researcher's theoretical or clinical background. In Mr R's story I was able to identify evidence both in his account and from clinical practice that his wife's lack of motivation and anger could be symptoms of depression, a treatable illness. For this reason I was inclined to absolve Ms R rather than hold her blameworthy. In addition, Mr R seems to say that he is sending his wife to the nursing home *because of* her anger and lack of motivation – is he punishing her or protecting himself?

The workings of Mr R's heart are closed to us. It is not possible for the reader, or perhaps even for Mr R, to know those secrets. His frequent repetitions hint that his heart may be less adamant than his rhetoric – Mr R does indeed protest a great deal. On the other hand, the relentless consistency of his story could be interpreted as evidence that he must protect his carefully fabricated and fragile sense of himself as 'fine and dandy' at almost any price.

In conclusion, the narrative researcher must constantly overread, find the secrets, show them, and yet resist the impulse to impose solutions that artificially reduce or foreclose inconsistency. The work of the narrative researcher is to find and to show, not to solve. Narrative researchers and practicing nurses who wish to be reliable witnesses to stories must, paradoxically, relinquish their need for rational solutions in service of the greater goal of fidelity to the stories with which they have been entrusted.

Note

1. First person pronoun in the remainder of this chapter refers to author Ayres.

References

Ayres, L. (2000a) Narratives of family caregiving: Four story types. *Research in Nursing and Health* **23**: 359–71.

Ayres, L. (2000b) Narratives of family caregiving: the process of making meaning. *Research in Nursing and Health* **23**: 424–34.

Ayres, L. & Poirier, S. (1996) Virtual text and the growth of meaning in qualitative analysis. *Research in Nursing and Health* **19**: 163–9.

Booth, W.C. (1983) *The Rhetoric of Fiction*, 2nd edn. Chicago: University of Chicago Press (first published in 1961).

Boykin, A. & Schoenhofer, S.O. (1991) Story as link between nursing practice, ontology, epistemology. *IMAGE: Journal of Nursing Scholarship* **23**: 245–8.

Brooks, P. (1984) *Reading for the Plot*. Cambridge, MA: Harvard University Press.

Bruner, J. (1986) *Actual Minds, Possible Worlds*. Cambridge, MA: Harvard University Press.

Coffey, A. & Atkinson, P. (1996) *Making Sense of Qualitative Data*. Thousand Oaks, CA: Sage.

Culler, J. (1981) *The Pursuit of Signs*. London: Routledge & Kegan Paul.

Iser, W. (1980) The reading process: a phenomenological approach. In J. Tompkins (ed.) *Reader-response Criticism*. Baltimore, MD: The Johns Hopkins University Press, pp. 50–69. Reprinted from W. Iser (1974) *The Implied Reader: Patterns in Communication in Prose from Bunyan to Becket*. Baltimore, MD: The Johns Hopkins University Press, pp. 274–99.

Kavanaugh, K. & Ayres, L. (1998) 'Not as bad as it could have been': Assessing and mitigating harm during research interviews on sensitive topics. *Research in Nursing and Health* **21**: 91–7.

Kermode, F. (1981) Secrets and narrative sequence. In W.J.T. Mitchell (ed.) *On Narrative*. Chicago: University of Chicago Press, pp. 79–97.

Knafl, K.A. & Ayres, L. (1996) Managing large data sets in family research. *Journal of Family Nursing* **2**: 350–64.

Lieblich, A., Tuval-Mashiach, R. & Zilber, T. (1998) *Narrative Research*. Thousand Oaks, CA: Sage.

Lincoln, Y.S. & Guba, E.G. (1985) *Naturalistic Inquiry*. Thousand Oaks, CA: Sage.

Miles, M.B. & Huberman, A.M. (1994) *Qualitative Data Analysis*, 2nd edn. Thousand Oaks, CA: Sage.

Mishler, E.G. (1986) *Research Interviewing*. Cambridge, MA: Harvard University Press.

Phillips, L.R., Morrison, E., Steffl, B., Young, M.C., Cromwell, S.L. & Russell, C.K. (1995) Effects of situational context and interactional process on the quality of family caregiving. *Research in Nursing & Health* **18**: 205–16.

Poirier, S. & Ayres, L. (1997) Endings, secrets, and silences: overreading in narrative inquiry. *Research in Nursing and Health* **20**: 551–7.

Polkinghorne, D.E. (1988) *Narrative Knowing and the Human Sciences.* Albany, NY: State University of New York Press.

Sandelowski, M. (1993) Rigor or rigor mortis: the problem of rigor in qualitative research revisited. *Advances in Nursing Science* **16**: 1–8.

Texts

'One ought to begin an analysis of power from the ground up, at the level of tiny local events where battles are unwittingly enacted by players who do not know what they are doing.' (Hacking, 1986: 28)

'Language is not a system of signs that represent. Rather, language appears as discourse, a material practice which systematically forms that of which it speaks.' (Deetz, 1992: 31)

Part IV explores approaches to researching the discursive relations which help order health care and nursing. Professional policy as well as many nursing theorists and researchers treat nurses as accountable individuals who can unproblematically decide how to act, and what to privilege. The chapters that follow offer an approach to research which helps illuminate not just how nurses and other people involved in health care work are not individuals able to simply choose how they think and act. Rather, the subjects of research emerge as positioned by their embeddedness in the societies in which they act. The authors show how this embeddedness and positioning can be illuminated through attention to discourse as those material practices which keep the world in order.

The texts with which the chapters are concerned have been generated in different ways: some texts derive from the transcription of interview data while others derive from documents and records, or from the recording of conversations as they 'naturally' occur in fieldwork settings. The term 'text' helps indicate that the text is made up of *interpretations*, which require further interpretation or 'reading'. It also indicates that language is not being taken at face value, as simply representing 'an absent, to be recalled object' (Deetz, 1992). Rather, textual analysis explores the cultural and historical definitions embedded in language which enable social organisation. Language is thus considered as made up of *systems of distinction*. Critically, however, not all systems of distinction are equal: some distinctions (and the people that articulate them) seem to have more authority than others, so that it is the constitutive effects of texts, and the tension between different textual representations of reality, which are of interest in the following chapters. Specifically, then, the authors attend to how language, as systems of distinction, classification and identity are produced, but not as the description of 'natural divisions', rather as articulations which have 'distinct political effect' (Deetz, 1992: 29).

References

Deetz, S. (1992) Disciplinary power in the modern corporation. In M. Alvesson and H. Willmott (eds) *Critical Management Studies*. London: Sage.

Hacking, I. (1986) The archaeology of Foucault. In Couzens Hoy (ed.) *Foucault: A Critical Reader*. Oxford: Basil Blackwell.

CHAPTER 8

Discourse analysis, ideology and professional practice

Michael Traynor

Many different approaches to understanding and interpreting talk and text go under the name of discourse analysis. Linguists, theologians and social scientists 'do discourse analysis', but their interests, theoretical bases and products can be quite different. In this chapter I want to do a number of things: first, set out a simple schema of some different approaches to discourse analysis used within the social sciences and linguistics. I will then discuss some examples of its use in analysis of health care settings, and within studies of nursing, midwifery and health visiting. The following part of the chapter will examine one approach to discourse analysis, an approach influenced by post-structuralism, and I will give an example of this approach in action. Without wishing to devalue any other approach, I will argue that this theoretical orientation can alert us to some dangers inherent in a discourse analytic approach if it is taken as a way either of accounting for intention or of presenting a stable or undeceived picture of the world, one that is able to perceive the reality beyond ideology.

Discourse analysis: a dual development

Before I attempt to untangle some of the different strands of activity that go under the name of discourse analysis, it would seem wise to agree on some definition of that overused term 'discourse'. At its most general level, discourse can be understood as any system of signs, whether spoken, written or otherwise. I say 'otherwise' because it is possible to 'read' town planning or architecture, for example, as signifiers of political values and practices (who is allowed proximity to whom, who is isolated, what does the colonnade of a Renaissance hospital, where patients are accommodated on the edges of a busy town square, say about beliefs about sickness and community?). Some use the term a little more specifically, so, for example a phrase such as 'medical discourse' implies an organised and more or less self-conscious system of concepts and language which reflects and is supported by an institutional base. Some while ago, Parker set out certain characteristics of discourse and, importantly, questioned the distinction between 'discourse' and 'reality'.

> 'Discourses do not simply describe the social world, they categorise it, they bring phenomena into sight... Once an object has been elaborated in a discourse, it is difficult not to refer to it as if it were real.' (Parker, 1992: 4–5)

Others, as I will show later, find little ground on which to draw any separation between discourse and whatever is outside of discourse.

Parker offers seven criteria for distinguishing discourses: a discourse is realised in texts, it is about objects, it contains subjects (simply put, the 'subject' who speaks or writes and the 'subject' the discourse is addressed to), it is a coherent system of meanings, it refers to other discourses, it reflects on its own way of speaking, and is historically located. In addition a discourse often supports institutions, reproduces power relationships and has ideological effects (Parker, 1992). Discourses are at work in texts, but texts, for Parker, are not merely written and spoken. Rather they are any form of construction that can be given an interpretative gloss. So, for example, the city architecture that I mentioned earlier, can be understood as a text.

What is discourse analysis?

Discourse analysis, then, at its most broad, is the analysis and interpretation of the operation of these signs as they relate to communicative practices between humans. The various practices that go under the name of discourse analysis have tended to develop within two separate, but not entirely unconnected, disciplinary areas. A catalogue search at my university library for 'discourse analysis' will send the reader scurrying on two distinct journeys. One is to the fourth floor of the North Wing to works on Social Sciences, theology and biblical studies. The other major journey is over to the South Wing, fifth floor, to studies of rhetoric, oral communication and speech pathology. The separation is not entirely transparent, because you would also find sociologist David Silverman's book on the father of conversation analysis, Harvey Sacks (Silverman, 1998), in this second location. A key work on discourse analysis, Teun A. van Dijk's *Discourse Studies: A Multidisciplinary Introduction*, is organised in two volumes: *Discourse as Structure and Process* (Dijk 1997a) and *Discourse as Social Interaction* (Dijk, 1997b). The first volume focuses on the analysis of verbal structures and cognitive processes; the second on discourse as interaction in society and to some extent this reflects the disciplinary and topological separation I have just described.

Each field is diverse and it is all too easy to generalise about either, so it is with hesitation that I suggest that the study of discourse within linguistics tends to have as its aim the discovery of communicative practices and principles from the study of speech data. In this field, some linguists do not work with 'naturally occurring data', but rather set up specific experiments. The work of Gillian Brown from the Research Centre for English and Applied Linguistics, University of Cambridge, typifies a particular type of analysis which is 'an investigation of the comprehension process'. In one piece of her research, she asks one set of subjects to explain features and routes on a map to a second set of subjects, and tape records and analyses the result (Brown, 1998). These studies do not make connections between such interactions and larger political or cultural practices. Also, while certainly not philosophically naive, some of this work appears to proceed from the assumption that language is a resource used more or less freely, by more or less fully conscious, autonomous individuals – a philosophical position that has been strongly critiqued over the past 30 years. Some linguists, however, would argue that this issue is intentionally side-stepped and that this is a strength of their work, rather than a naivety (Rendle-Short, personal communication).

Harvey Sacks, in many senses founded conversation analysis in the mid to late 1960s. His intention was to build up an understanding of social life from an investigation of actual linguistic events (Silverman, 1998). Although there are differences between his approach and the ethnomethodology developed by Garfinkel, like his contemporary he was concerned to investigate how people accomplish 'being ordinary' and the rules that speakers attend to in actual examples of talk. Such concerns clearly straddle the division between linguistics and the social sciences.

Discourse analysis within the social sciences tends to link analysis of talk or text, to social structures and sociological theory, sometimes to local hegemonic processes and structures or other political struggles and a field of critical discourse analysis has developed. For some critical discourse analysts, social life is a practice and any practice generates representations of that practice (Chouliaraki and Fairclough, 1999).[1] Chouliaraki and Fairclough (1999) argue that many practices involve struggles for power and closure that never completely succeed and always give rise to resistance. The issues of power and resistance are of particular interest to critical discourse analysts. Lupton (1995: 302) asks similar questions:

> 'How do individuals take up, negotiate, or resist discourse and how is resistance generated and sustained? What are the constraints to taking up subject positions? How are the individuals interpellated, or "hailed" by discourses, how do they recognise themselves within?'

Discourse analysis for these researchers involves the documentation and investigation of these processes based on analysis of conversational data or other 'texts'. The link between discursive practice and ideology is explicit within certain approaches undertaken in France. Michel Pêcheau and colleagues have adopted a particular analytical tool to empirically investigate ideological practices that were proposed by Marxist Louis Althusser (Pêcheau, 1995). So, to summarise: approaches to discourse analysis can be arranged in terms of how interested the analyst is in making connections between individual interaction or utterance and larger political and structural forces. However, there is another dimension along which we can place studies of discourse, and this is to do with the analyst's ideas about the human subject and its relationship to language.

The question of the subject

Structuralism originated at the beginning of the twentieth century in linguistics and went on to influence a range of disciplines, particularly in Europe, notably anthropology and psychoanalysis. Simply put, it challenged two assumptions about language: that the meaning of words corresponds to the objects outside of language to which they refer, and that the human subject, who is a rational and conscious entity, assigns these meanings to words and assembles them in order to communicate ideas. Structuralism argued that the system of language provided the range of conceptual categories that were available to individuals (De Saussure, 1996) and post-structuralism went on to suggest that even what we understand as human individuality was a result of available ways of thinking and talking about the human subject (Foucault, 1972). Some discourse analysts, understanding language from these structuralist and post-structuralist perspectives, which tend to decentre the human subject, criticise 'orthodox linguistics' for its adherence to a philosophically discredited – they would argue – understanding of the human subject:

> 'Orthodox linguistics is very much a product of modernity – [it pictures] the centred rational subject as dipping into the resources of language in order to convey a meaning which is created and controlled by that individual subject.' (Williams, 1999: 5)

Analysts working from this perspective would tend to foreground the system of language itself when investigating the effect of discourse, rather than the subject who is speaking or listening.

These differences of interest and approach can be represented on the two dimensions shown in Fig. 8.1, which I owe, in part, to Alvesson and Karreman (2000). In fact, the two dimensions cannot really be considered orthogonal because analysts who are concerned to foreground linguistic structures may well also emphasise political and other social structures within their analysis.

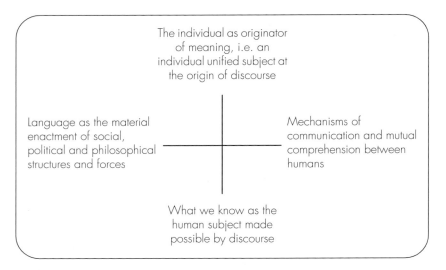

The individual as originator
of meaning, i.e. an
individual unified subject at
the origin of discourse

Language as the material
enactment of social,
political and philosophical
structures and forces

Mechanisms of
communication and mutual
comprehension between
humans

What we know as the
human subject made
possible by discourse

Fig. 8.1 Two dimensions of discourse analysis (based on Alvesson and Karreman, 2000).

Discourse analysis in health care

If we can think of discourse analysis as having two aspects, roughly corresponding to points near each end of the horizontal axis of Fig. 8.1, then both have a great deal to offer to the study and understanding of health care. Analysts who focus on conversation analysis, such as Silverman, can show us how clinicians and their patients each attempt to establish their identities and roles, sometimes in a kind of agonistic interchange. Silverman's work (Silverman, 1987) on consultations between paediatric cardiologists and the parents of children with cardiac malformations are classics of this approach because they show us the complexity of the clinical consultation and how clinicians, through verbal resources, attempt to present certain ways of understanding a child and his or her health problems in a particular light, and sometimes how parents resist this persuasion. (In fact, this work of Silverman combines both approaches.) Others have looked at aspects of nursing interactions. For example, Susan Sefi has examined how health visitors attempt to manage giving child care advice to their clients (Heritage and Sefi, 1992).

Those analysts who wish to link analysis of talk or text to political and philosophical structures have also much to contribute to a political and sociological understanding of the changing public sector and the professional cultures within it. I have attempted this in some of my work, and a presentation of some of this follows.

Nurses and a discourse of moral agency

Discourse analysis can show how different groups in the health care arena represent their activities, and the activities of others, and can help to reveal the mechanisms of political and professional struggle. Apparently casual talk can show the operation of powerful discourses that derive from broad historical and cultural forces. In work which I carried out looking at the effects of a major reorganisation of the UK National Health Service (Traynor, 1996, 1999), I was able to compare the talk of groups of front-line community nurses with that of senior managers. Each group discursively created its own subjectivity partly in relation to a constructed subjectivity of the other, which acted to intensify its own position. Unfortunately, I have space only to describe how one of these groups achieved this. My theoretical position is that broad cultural discourse makes available certain 'subject positions' through which individuals must understand, present and perform their own 'identity'. The nurses tended to call on an available discourse of the self-sacrificing moral agent and contrasted this with managers whom they described as detached from direct involvement in physical and emotional reality and more oriented towards supposedly more abstract activities such as financial management.

My source of data was not conversation but 886 remarks written by nurses from four NHS trusts on the open-ended section of a questionnaire which I distributed three times, at yearly intervals. More background and methodological details can be found elsewhere in the original accounts of the research I alluded to above. I present here a summary of one possibility for analysis.

I argue that the nurses' broad subject position is built up through a number of moves (these discursive moves are not necessarily conscious). The first is to reposition their activity away from the purely occupational to the personal vocational.

These two discourses (the occupational, associated with financial remuneration and bureaucratic structures, and the vocational, linked with higher-order human rewards) have to pre-exist and each be valued in particular ways for such a move to be possible and have an effect:

> 'Each day I aim to do my job to 100% of my capabilities to ensure my patients' well-being and happiness, and then return home to do the same for the rest of my family.' (Practice nurse)

The moral orientation of their work was made possible by constructing the patient as bringing a moral state, that of need, to the encounter. Nurses conveyed a sense of urgency regarding this need, yet it also appeared, paradoxically, to be something that was detected and defined by nurses:

> 'Approx. $\frac{1}{3}$ of my caseload comprises of families of concern who need extra HV support and it is a constant struggle to provide them with the professional support/guidance which they need and are entitled to.' (Health visitor)

> 'As a student I have more opportunity to spend longer time with patients/families, time that THEY NEED.' (District nursing student, emphasis in original)

The next move begins to present the nurse as frustrated rather than achieving satisfaction from this moral activity. This can have the effect of raising the value of the activity because it is not self-interested:

> 'Nurses desperately trying to maintain a high standard of care to patients...' (District nurse)

> '[I am] always aiming to offer the patients in the care of my team a high standard of quality care. I am now struggling to continue my standard of care.' (District nurse)

This self-sacrifice is pictured as exploitation. This avoids a presentation of moral reluctance, which would be problematic because it would undercut a moral stance. The position of self-sacrifice could also augment the injustice of what they described as their exploitation because their moral orientation and sensitivity rendered them highly vulnerable to abuse:

'Nurses are sick of being used and abused by the system.' (Staff nurse)

'The worker can have given a lifetime of commitment ... and at the end of the day it is totally forgotten.' (Health visitor)

This construction of a 'moral high ground' enabled nurses to denigrate the consideration for finances which they associated with management:

'The world of business has definitely taken over, and as well as not giving as much time to the patients as we would like, there is a lack of caring for us as the carers.' (District nurse)

'Numbers, finances and balancing books [are] becoming more important than people. The organisation doesn't really CARE for its workforce.' (Health visitor, emphasis in original)

What I have tried to do is to argue that discourses at large are available to be drawn upon by groups seeking to define and strengthen their position and identity at times of conflict. Close examination of texts can provide evidence for this process. I would like to emphasise that these analyses are not aimed at a discrediting of nurses, or 'exposing' 'real' motivation because such post-structuralist theories do not imply that these processes are conscious or freely chosen.

Warnings and qualifications: discourse, ideology and intention

The nurses' and managers' texts have ideological effects. Their words can be seen as ideological self-presentations, working with the material of caring, cash, motivation and modernity, arranging and presenting these materials in ways that have certain effects, tell certain stories, emphasise, perhaps, the centrality of their respective positions or subjectivities. However, there is little that is 'raw' about this material. There is no reality to be seen beyond the mist of ideology; no original 'care' or even 'cash' that can be isolated to stand apart from how we construct and employ them; no signified referred to unambiguously by the signifiers of nurses and managers. As post-structuralists argue, one signifier leads to another in endless fashion. So 'ideological', if its utterance implies a contrasting world of reality, is not the best word. The term 'discursive' has been used to avoid that sense that there can be privileged access, for some, to reality. Let me clarify this point. When I say that, in a sense, it is not helpful to talk of 'real caring' I do not mean to suggest that caring is not experienced by people every day or that I do not personally value 'caring' as a characteristic. I mean that what we might mean by the term, its significance to us, the uses we put it to, cannot be apprehended apart from our own culture's ways of thought, whether explicit or otherwise. Historians of nursing, Nutting and Dock, were aware of the importance of this kind of context when, drawing upon the work of Russian zoologist Kropotkin, they constructed 'caring' as the key to human evolutionary success and in the process elevated the importance of nurses considerably (Nutting and Dock, 1907: 6). Many other nursing writers since then have promoted a similar understanding of caring (Leininger, 1978; Benner and Wrubel, 1989; Morse and Field, 1996).

But there are two further qualifications. The first is to do with intention. The shift from a concern with the individual to the organising life of structures is a key move in structuralist thought. Literary theorist Eagleton makes this explicit:

> 'The confident bourgeois belief that the isolated individual subject was the fount and origin of all meaning took a sharp knock [with structuralism]: language pre-dated the individual, and was much less his or her product than he or she was the product of it. Meaning was not "natural", a question of just looking and seeing . . . One result of structuralism, then, is the "decentring" of the individual subject, who is no longer to be regarded as the source or end of meaning.' (Eagleton, 1983: 107/104)

As I said, I would not want to claim that the discursive effects that I have drawn attention to in my account of nurses are necessarily fully conscious or intended by them. I would argue, instead, that certain discourses and subject positions are so available at certain moments in history that individuals almost cannot help but adopt them, particularly when defending positions they feel to be under threat. In a slightly more agentic explanation, Callon describes processes of 'enrolment' of interests or 'translation' where one group attempts to align the interests of another group to its own (Callon *et al.*, 1986). Joanna Latimer has explored the notions of enrolment and translation as partial explanations for nursing's uptake of the nursing process and managerialist projects (Latimer, 1995). She suggests that while nurses find something within these discourses of use to them, they are inevitably and perhaps unwittingly drawn onto the discursive ground implicit in these projects, believing them to be largely 'neutral' technologies.

It would be a mistake, however, to seek an origin of the broad notions of caring and rational efficiency in particular groups, in, for example, professional nursing bodies or government departments. Without claiming that these notions represent fundamental human structures, their genealogy is long and complex and perhaps the best we can do is to observe that certain groups have found it advantageous to become associated with them.

Discourse and stability

So far, I have shown a picture of a group that self-consciously places itself in contrast to some other. There is however a rather simplistic aesthetic satisfaction to be found in this structure that also has unwitting political effects by maintaining the representation of unity and stability of these two objects – nurses and managers.

The identification of nurses involved in care delivery with a moral agency and of managers with 'rationality' does not do justice to either the ambiguity nor the instability of the subject positions adopted by each group. Such a presentation tends to homogenise the two groups. It ignores those occasions when nurses drew upon utilitarian notions, for example by arguing that the money spent on 'another glossy brochure from the Government' (field notes nursing staff meeting, December 1993) could have funded a number of extra nursing posts. The nurses here display a wicked ability to jump out, for a moment, of any stable identity that we might wish to place them in. Also, characterising the utilitarian discourse adopted by managers as an expression of rationality fails to take account of utilitarianism as an approach devised to answering essentially moral problems, such as how to use (supposedly) scarce resources. It is an approach, however, which has been seen as misguided

(MacIntyre, 1985). While the presentation of nurses' texts given in this chapter remains a useful account of the effect of powerful discourses and provides certain aesthetic satisfaction, there is a danger that such a presentation reproduces the very discursive identities that these groups are enacting, colluding in their desire for stability and unity of identity, an identity achieved, as I have suggested, by the fierce exclusion of the other.

No account of an object can do justice to its instability, yet signifiers too are subject to drift. Derrida argues that within the western tradition of what he calls 'logocentrism', with its 'metaphysical longing for origin and ideals', speech has been privileged and writing seen as a kind of corrupt activity, parasitic upon speech. Part of the very structure of the written word is that it is separable from the present, the context of its inscription and is citable in new contexts. However, Derrida, seeking to overturn this dualism, claims that even speech is subject to similar 'drifts' in meaning through the possibility of its appearance in different contexts:

> 'Every sign, linguistic or nonlinguistic, spoken or written, … as a small or large unity, can be cited, put between quotation marks; thereby it can break with every given context, and engender infinitely new contexts in an absolutely nonsaturable fashion. This does not suppose that the mark is valid outside its context, but on the contrary that there are only contexts without any centre of absolute anchoring. This citationality, duplication, or duplicity, this iterability of the mark is not an accident or an anomaly, but is that … without which a mark could no longer even have a so-called 'normal' functioning. What would a mark be that one could not cite? And whose origin could not be lost on the way?' (Derrida, 1982: 320–21)

But what of intention? Intention cannot be considered as a single fixed point of origin:

> 'When questioned about the implications of an utterance I may quite routinely include in my intention implications that had never previously occurred to me. My intention is the sum of further explanations I might give when questioned on any point and is thus less an origin than a product, less a delimited

content than an open set of discursive possibilities ... intentions do not ... suffice to determine meaning; context must be mobilised.' (Culler, 1983: 127–8)

In other words, an utterance acts in different ways depending on the context in which it is placed. Intentional, original and metaphysically privileged meaning, if such a thing exists, cannot set a boundary around all future or possible meanings. How then can we understand the task of the reader of literature, historical documents, the transcripts of interviews with NHS managers or the status of any human utterance or mark? Deconstruction offers the suggestion of an aporia, or impasse, a double movement between two opposed yet simultaneous approaches:

'If we say that the meaning of a work is the reader's response, we nevertheless show, in our descriptions of response, that interpretation is an attempt to discover meaning in the text. If we propose some other decisive determinant of meaning, we discover that the factors deemed crucial are subject to interpretation in the same way as the text itself and thus defer the meaning they determine.' (Culler, 1983: 132–3)

Within the signifier then, we might say that there is an unavoidable, and unsatisfiable, desire for the (lost) original and origin.

Any account is thus a simplification, and just that, an account, but we are left with the problematic relationship between the presentation of discourse analysis and the 'objects' of inquiry.

Desire for 'the real thing'

Philosopher Richard Rorty offers one way out of this problem, suggesting that we stop thinking of inquiry as seeking a representation of reality but rather as a continual recontextualisation of our present beliefs. He argues that, at our point in history, still influenced by modernism, we have yet to escape completely the idea that inquiry is a matter of

'finding out the nature of something which lies outside the web of beliefs and desires. There still lingers some sense in which the object of inquiry ... has a context of its own, a context which is privileged by virtue of it being the object's rather than the enquirer's.' (Rorty, 1991: 96)

In reply to questions about objects and their contexts, Rorty would claim that all objects are always already contextualised. They all come with contexts attached.

Another approach to this problem might be to adopt some literary theorists' rejection of the traditional distinction between the text and the critical work which comments upon that text (de Man, 1979). For some, the poetic or literary work has no sacrosanct and unique autonomy, nor has the work of criticism a privileged status over and above the works it critiques (Norris, 1991). The critical enterprise itself is bound to use the same persuasive techniques as the texts it attempts to unravel. In the same way, the account that I have given claims no privileged access to truth about the texts I have analysed and attempted to deconstruct. This work is ultimately rhetorical, as is the case, I would argue, for any inquiry that, unlike this one, claims access to a metaphysical grounding, whether that grounding be located in scientific methodology or in the privilege of direct experience or insight.

Desire for identity

Discourse provides possibilities for identity, as I have suggested in my claim that nurses and managers adopted certain subject positions, subject positions that are, like language itself, culturally, irresistibly almost, available. From this theoretical point of view, we might understand identity as largely a discursive and historically contingent achievement rather than a pre-existing aspect of human autonomy. Cixous sees modern western habits of thought as responsible not only for notions of individual freedom and autonomy but also for a potentially harmful rejection of otherness:

'Ours is an era [where] ... a phobia of non-identity has spread and nations like individuals are infected with this neurosis, this pain, this fear of non-recognition, where each constructs, erects his auto-identification, less out of intimate reflection than out of a system of rejection and hatred. The Serb says: I am no Croatian; to be Croatian is to be non-Serb. And each affirms him- or herself as distinct, as unique and non other, as though there were room only for one and not for two, as if two and otherness were forbidden.' (Cixous, 1993: 202–3)

I have argued that nurses, whether fully intentionally or not, constructed their identity partially by attributing certain discourses to the other group and by seeking to understand and present themselves through the exclusion of those discourses. Everything that can be, however spuriously, associated with the other loses its legitimacy and provides further material for the construction of one's own group's identity. It is possible to see the expulsion of an excluded element, 'a scapegoat charged with the evil of which the community duly constituted can then purge itself, a purge which will finally exonerate that community' as an essential move in the continuous formation of any community (Kristeva, 1996). It is possible, therefore, to see a desire for identity enacted in discourse.

Summary

Different approaches to discourse analysis exist and many have a valuable contribution to make to inquiry into health service provision. I have focused on one approach that is influenced by post-structuralism and presented some discussions about representation in discourse from this perspective.

Perhaps the discourses of nurses that I have discussed in this chapter (and of managers which I have not discussed) can be understood as enacting a desire for coherence, identity and solidarity partly through a connection to different historical projects or historical communities (real or imagined). It is this identification that can help to make the positions and arguments of different groups more powerful.

Discourse (in the post-structuralist sense) masquerades as the natural. It disguises its own artifice. However, from a post-structuralist perspective at least, it would be a mistake to look for some reality that is apprehended once we have escaped discourse – if it were possible to do that. Perhaps the discourse analyst can be understood as facing a temptation to 'possess the real' in his or her descriptions while at the same time trying to avoid claiming any privileged position. I have proposed that Richard Rorty's under-standing of inquiry as recontextualisation rather than representa-tion, and post-structuralism's rejection of the hierarchical distinction between the text and the critique, provide two stances towards our activities that can help us, as discourse analysts, avoid this contradiction. The usefulness of discourse analysis is that it can make visible the workings of text, talk or other systems of signs and thus make it easier to understand their effects and even challenge them.

For me, the most impressive examples of discourse analysis are those which combine meticulous scrutiny of signs (such as the sign-making going on within conversation) with a sophisticated philo-sophical and political analysis. Both are immensely useful in the study of illness, health and health care.

Note

1. Harvey Sacks argued something similar, suggesting that human inter-action was like a process with two outputs: one was the interaction, the other was a constant simultaneous commentary on that interaction (Silverman, 1998).

References

Alvesson, M. and Karreman, D. (2000) Varieties of discourse: on the study of organisations through discourse analysis. *Human Relations* 53 (9): 1125–49.

Benner, P. and Wrubel, J. (1989) *The Primacy of Caring: Stress and Coping in Health and Illness*. California: Addison-Wesley.

Brown, G. (1998) *Speakers, Listeners and Communication: Explorations in Discourse Analysis*. Cambridge: Cambridge University Press.

Callon, M., Law, J. & Rip, A. (eds) (1986) *Mapping the Dynamics of Science and Technology*. Basingstoke: Macmillan.

Chouliaraki, L. and Fairclough, N. (1999) *Discourse Analysis in Late Modernity: Rethinking Critical Discourse Analysis*. Edinburgh: Edin-burgh University Press.

Cixous, H. (1993) We who are free, are we free? *Critical Inquiry* 19 (2): 201.

Culler, J. (1983) *On Deconstruction: Theory and Criticism after Structuralism*. London: Routledge.

de Man, P. (1979) *Allegories of Reading: figurative language in Rousseau, Nietzsche, Rilke, and Proust*. New Haven, CT: Yale University Press.

De Saussure, F. (1996) Selections from the Course in General Linguistics. In R. Kearney & M. Rainwater (eds) *The Continental Philosophy Reader*. London: Routledge, pp. 291–304.

Derrida, J. (1982) *Signature Event Context. Margins of Philosophy*. Hemel Hempstead: Harvester Wheatsheaf, pp. 307–30.

Dijk, T.A. v. (ed.) (1997a) *Discourse Studies: A Multidisciplinary Introduction. Vol. 1. Discourse as Structure and Process*. London, Sage.

Dijk, T.A. v. (ed.) (1997) *Discourse Studies: A Multidisciplinary Introduction. Vol. 2. Discourse as Social Interaction*. London, Sage.

Eagleton, T. (1983) *Literary Theory: An Introduction*. Oxford: Blackwell.

Foucault, M. (1972) *The Archaeology of Knowledge*. London: Routledge.

Heritage, J. and Sefi, S. (1992) Dilemmas of advice: aspects of the delivery and reception of advice in interactions between health visitors and first time mothers. In P. Drew and J. Heritage (eds) *Talk at Work*. Cambridge: Cambridge University Press.

Kristeva, J. (1996) Women's time. In R. Kearney & M. Rainwater (eds) *The Continental Philosophy Reader*. London: Routledge, pp. 378–401.

Latimer, J. (1995) The nursing process re-examined: diffusion or translation? *Journal of Advanced Nursing* **22**: 213–20.

Leininger, M. (1978) *Transcultural Nursing. Concepts, Theories and Practices*. New York: Wiley.

Lupton, D. (1995) D & S forum: Postmodernism and critical discourse analysis. *Discourse and Society* **6** (2): 301–4.

MacIntyre, A. (1985) *After Virtue. A Study in Moral Theory*. London: Duckworth.

Morse, J. & Field, P. (1996) *Nursing Research: The Application of Qualitative Approaches*. London: Chapman & Hall.

Norris, C. (1991) *Deconstruction: Theory and Practice*. London: Routledge.

Nutting, M. & Dock, L. (1907) *A History of Nursing: The Evolution of Nursing Systems from the Earliest Times to the Foundation of the First English and American Training Schools*. London: G.P. Putnam's & Sons.

Parker, I. (1992) *Discourse Dynamics: Critical Analysis for Social and Individual Psychology*. London: Routledge.

Pêcheau, M. (1995) *Automatic Discourse Analysis*. Amsterdam: Radopi.

Rorty, R. (1991) Inquiry as recontextualisation: an anti-dualist account of interpretation. Objectivity, relativism and truth. *Philosophical Papers* **1**: 93–110.

Silverman, D. (1987) *Communication and Medical Practice: Social Relations in the Clinic*. London: Sage.

Silverman, D. (1998) *Harvey Sacks: Social Science and Conversation Analysis*. Cambridge: Cambridge University Press.

Traynor, M. (1996) A literary approach to managerial discourse after the NHS reforms. *Sociology of Health and Illness* **18**(3): 315–40.

Traynor, M. (1999) *Managerialism and Nursing: Beyond Profession and Oppression*. London: Routledge.

Williams, G. (1999) *French Discourse Analysis: The Method of Post-structuralism*. London: Routledge.

CHAPTER 9

Words are powerful tools: discourse analytic explanations of nursing practice

Trudy Rudge

In this chapter, I offer an approach to studying nursing which brings together ethnography with discourse analysis and uses ideas deriving from social and psychoanalytic theory to discuss nurse and patient interactions.

Exploring common intimacies inhering to nursing work, the approach focuses on how nurses and patients interact, and explicates how these interactions are socially constructed *as well as* individualised. In attending to the implicit *and* explicit beliefs and knowledges which underpin these nursing occasions, the approach illuminates how nurses accomplish much more than the usual representations of nursing work would have us believe. Specifically, by analysing talk and interaction as involving more than the mere words that are said (Fairclough, 1992, 1995; Burman & Parker, 1993; Silverman, 1993), the analysis explicates how the words used, and the meanings attributed to them make certain thoughts and actions possible (Foucault, 1970; Fairclough, 1992). In addition, the approach helps explain why nurses might be engaged in practice in the ways they are, and why many aspects of their accomplishments remain invisible to mainstream research methodologies in nursing.

To exemplify the approach, the chapter draws on an ethnography of wound care (Rudge, 1997). For nursing, the care of wounds is widespread. It entails occasions where a nurse and a patient interact with a common focus, that is, getting a wound healed. Wound care may also entail nurses educating patients/clients to take over the care of the wound from the nurse. It is an aspect of medical work which nurses pride themselves in as experts. However, wound care is often represented as if it consists of practices which are merely standardised, based on evidence derived far from nurse–patient interactions. In contrast, by stressing wound care as *produced* through nurse–patient interaction, the current approach asserts the relationship between nurse and patient as a main feature of wound care practice. By asserting this emphasis, wound care emerges as much more than the application of technical procedures for the healing of wounds. In addition, by laying the analysis of how nurses work with patients' bodies alongside formal representations of wound care work, the extent to which wound care emerges as a discursively constructed aspect of nursing which is taken for granted (or 'naturalised') can emerge. That is, while wound care practices *appear* natural, the approach to analysis offered here helps us to understand them differently: by making the complexity of wound care visible, that which is usually implicit about nursing work becomes explicit.

The analysis examines the discursive construction of wound care practices to expose the beliefs and knowledges which shape, constrain and make some ways of thinking and acting possible in caring for a wound, while excluding others. Thus wound care, which appears both physical and scientific, re-emerges as subject to the structuring effects of language and power. In figuring such an emergence it becomes obvious how words, whatever their textual source, are imbued with the power to influence and shape nursing practice. Central to this thinking is the understanding that words are not neutral in their effects; rather the choice of words, how the texts are constructed and what discursive influences are evident within them, construct these multiple realities. Thinking about language in this way also asserts that language does more than convey 'naturalised' meanings, exposing the influence of power relations in the everyday practices of nurses during wound care.

The chapter begins with an overview of the approach and the research context. It goes on to demonstrate the approach to analysis. First, by laying different accounts of wound care practice alongside each other I explicate how 'official' medical and nursing records are impoverished accounts which hide rather than show what nurses do. Second, I present analysis of two wound care occasions in which nurses and patients interact while undertaking a wound care dressing. The discussion and analysis of these instances of text, talk and practice provide examples of the forms of qualitative analysis that are possible with such data. The discussion and analysis of formal texts on wound care laid alongside the actual practice observations of talk and interaction emphasises how the official medical record erases nurses' practices. From the analysis of the interactions it is evident that wound care is a 'social' situation where competing interests are played out in an emotional situation, and that this situation remains absent from the official medical and nursing record texts. An analysis of the emotional import of skin, and the effects of its traumatisation, suggests that wound care is a nursing procedure whose emotional impact is minimised.

The research approach and context

The approach used in the study was ethnographic in its intent, with a discourse analytic approach to the analysis of the data derived from fieldwork in settings where burns and wound care were an acknowledged interest. The data collected was from settings and textual practices varying in their levels of formality. This approach to collection of data was to define a 'field' where wound and burns care was practised and they were a focus in spoken and written texts. This process of definition ensured that the study was situated in this procedure's most information-rich locations. Hence, observations and interviews occurred in a burns unit during wound care procedures, interviews with patients and nurses occurred after these dressings, with a final interview on discharge with the patients, as well as at the conclusion of the field work in the unit with the participating nurses.

In defining the field of 'interest', it was apparent that influences on wound care practices resided not only in the protocols for care of burns. These concerns were framed in the professional literature, pharmaceutical literature on wound dressing and wound care products, at wound care interest groups and workshops and during conferences where wound and/or burns care were a focus for the conference participants. Wound care practices are a source of considerable power and expertise in nursing, with many nurses considering themselves experts in diagnosis, treatment and healing of wounds (see Wicks, 1999). The professional forums where nurses discuss these issues were also a part of the study, and these included conferences, workshops for nurses to learn about wound healing and wound care product selection, pharmaceutical companies' literature on wound care (see Rudge, 1999), and professional journals and writing about wound care. These locations were also sources of valuable information about the professional milieu of this nursing practice.

However, nursing practice occurs within a field of knowledge about nursing itself. This meant that the literature explored for discursive effects on wound care included nursing theories and knowledges that acted as a source of caring practices. Such sources were found to include nursing theories about self-care, and approaches to organising care, such as nursing diagnoses. The source of this form of textual data in the unit came from a computerised care planning system which used 'units of care' deemed to be appropriate in burns care with time allocations and acuity ratings conceived as longer periods of time and intensity of work. That is, there were more units of care for those patients who required more care, and fewer for those who required less care from nurses. Hence, the number of pages for each 24-hour care plan reduced with the length of stay, or increased postoperatively when more care was required. These care plans did not remain with the medical record on discharge, but were instead kept for future reference for nurses within the unit.

Research context

The research focused on an Australian burns unit, which serviced a vast geographical area. Patients were admitted directly to the unit which comprised eight single rooms, an operating suite, a dressing room and bathroom that could be combined, and various service rooms for the operating suite and unit. Each of the five patients who agreed to participate in this study was admitted to the unit with an initial assessment that their burn comprised an area of greater than 25% and less than 50% of their body surface, to varying depths. They all required surgical debridement and grafting to obtain cover, although some areas such as their faces did not require grafting. All of the patients were men as there were no women admitted to the unit with this extent of burn during the 14 months of observational study. Such an event is not uncommon, with males being more likely to make up this group of patients.

There were 20 nursing staff employed on the unit at the time of the study, with 16 nurses agreeing to participate in either observation and/or interview. The nursing staff who did not participate were three nurses who were on regular night duty, and one nurse who did not agree to participate. The medical staff comprised two visiting specialists, two plastic surgery registrars, and a surgical intern who was rotated every three months. There was a clerical officer for the unit, a patient care attendant who stocked the rooms and the service areas, and two cleaners (these two women remained the same for the entire study) who are considered as integral to the team, maintaining the cleanliness of the rooms and the unit.

The phenomena under study were the interactions between patients and nurses during wound care procedures. Care of the burns wound makes up a considerable part of the care provided in such units. The extent of the burn in these cases meant that to clean the wound required the nurse to bathe the patient in bed, or, if walking, to shower him. The observations occurred in the bedroom or the bathroom, wherever the patient was to have their dressing attended to that day. The observations could take anything from 20 minutes to 3 hours, depending on the amount of graft, dressing and wound care required. I observed each patient at least three times a week during their hospitalisation (from five weeks to four months, with length of stay dependent on the area and degree of burn), interviewing them formally three times.

The nurses who agreed to participate were observed as they did the wound care procedure, and interviewed informally after this about what they thought was going on. Sometimes later in the study, the patient and nurse would talk informally about what happened, such conversations noted and recorded in the field notes along with the observations and the researcher's thoughts about the observation and interpretative comments. A final interview of all the nurses who had been observed occurred at the completion of the study. This interview explored their professional history, their learning on the unit, their beliefs about the care, and what they saw as being the characteristics of such nursing, its place in the organisation and any particular issues that they thought affected what happened in the unit.

In the larger study, data from interviews, observations, professional meetings and workshops, literature from pharmaceutical companies and professional journals were considered as part of the discursive field of power/knowledge that intersected with the nurses' and patients' interactions during wound care. Collation of this data into a framework for analysis proved to be a formidable task. However, in this chapter I explore the intersections in the 'field' of data collected specifically from the unit about patient care, and from occasions of wound care itself. Each patient had extensive medical records, nursing care plans (for each day of their stay), observations done during the wound care procedure, and interviews (both informal and formal). This chapter cannot do this justice, but it is hoped that exploring and analysing excerpts from the case notes, nursing care plans, and the nurses' practices themselves will show how such an ethnographic approach, wedded to a discourse analysis, brings into view the complex interplay of power relations and societal influences that impact on nursing practice.

'Daily dressing': the erasure of burns care

In this section I use various textual records from a patient's case notes and nursing care plan. Throughout this section, my focus will be on the location of the textual data as this reveals the power relations organising care, the manner of reporting, what is reported, and make some points about how all these aspects of textuality position nurses and patients in the official and off-the-record 'texts' of hospitalisation. These excerpts report on a patient's wound care after he had been for surgical debridement of some of his burns, harvesting of skin from a donor site on his leg, and application of this donor skin to his arms and flanks. These examples show the 'official' record of nurses' practices in the unit and are kept in the progress notes in the medical record. I provide some fuller description of this record from my observations of this dressing, and then show how this is recorded in the computerised nursing care plan which is used to organise patient care over a 24-hour period. These particular politics of recording are important because they signal how nursing work continues to be underestimated and easily 'forgotten' (Bowker & Star, 2000). More importantly, these politics are evidence of the practices of erasure under which nurses and patients interact during episodes of care.

In the unit where this study took place, the daily wound care needs of the patient were prescribed in a dressing book (outside of the official record) and in the nursing care plan for each patient (not kept in the medical record on discharge; see Bowker and Star, 2000). The following report headed 'Nursing', was in the patient's progress notes for his morning report the day after a surgical debridement of his burns:

> '*Wounds:* Bleeder stopped on R) arm. Both arms dressed in tulle and combine and splints. SSD [silver sulphadiazine] applied to back. 4/24 [four hourly] wet packs applied to L & R flank. Donors intact. 4/24 face care attended. Duoderm^{TM} on pressure sore on L) heel.'

This nursing note reports the dressings done, what is applied to particular areas, and the state of the donors and grafts. This is a technical summary of the wound care received by the patient on that day. His arms have been grafted, as have the burns on his flanks. His face still requires wound care to some of the areas with deeper burns and the areas around his ears that are slower to heal. At this stage the patient was resting in bed and his dressing was done in the morning in a process which lasted 2 hours, with an extra 30 minutes required for care of the unhealed burns on his face. Figure 9.1 is the wound care outlined in his nursing care plan.

This care plan 'unit of care' states that this is a large daily dressing, setting aside 90–180 minutes for its completion. The actual detail of what the dressing entails is not recorded here – instead it directs nurses to the off-the-record dressing book. The donor site care reports the type of product used to dress it, actions for nurses (that is, observe, reinforce, document, report). Moreover, while the note in his medical record is quite extensive, and my description of the dressing even longer, much of the nursing work in this unit was represented under the rather 'simple' umbrella of these words in the patients' records: 'daily dressing attended' or, 'Daily dressing ✓' or in the care plan 'Wound dressing – daily'. This form of notation in the official record of patient progress underscores how much of wound care is routinised and underdetermined in the work of the unit. For instance, the time taken for the dressing for this patient is

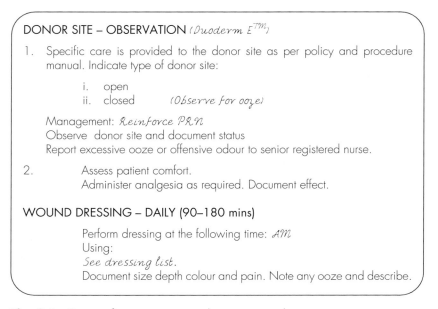

DONOR SITE – OBSERVATION *(Duoderm E^{TM})*

1. Specific care is provided to the donor site as per policy and procedure manual. Indicate type of donor site:

    i. open
    ii. closed   *(Observe for ooze)*

Management: *Reinforce PRN*
Observe donor site and document status
Report excessive ooze or offensive odour to senior registered nurse.

2.   Assess patient comfort.
    Administer analgesia as required. Document effect.

WOUND DRESSING – DAILY (90–180 mins)

    Perform dressing at the following time: *AM*
    Using:
    See dressing list.
    Document size depth colour and pain. Note any ooze and describe.

Fig. 9.1 Excerpts from a computerised nursing care plan.

two hours, with another half an hour for the face care. This is over one-quarter of the nurse's shift on the unit, and does not detail all the other work required for this patient over that time, or for other patients with similar needs. This is the time spent on the dressing alone. When such a notation, 'Daily dressing ✓', accomplishes the recording of this event in a medical record, the question remains, how can this stand adequately for such a process and what does such a diminishment accomplish?

As I have argued elsewhere (see Rudge, 1998), skin and bodies are spatial elements in the nursing practices of the burns unit. In accomplishing the work in such a unit, the 'things' (Sandelowski, 2000) worked with in the construction of the space of the dressing are the wound, 'skin' as graft, wound care dressing products, implements for doing dressings, and nurses' and patients' bodies. Within the social space (Lefebvre, 1991) built during a wound care procedure, the 'coverings' used to re-cover the patient's body are manipulated to result in the dressing of the patient's extensive wounds. However, through the process of standardisation of the recording of these activities in the official texts, the practices of nurses become represented as standardised, and indeed, expected to be standardised. Such standardisation achieves an erasure of the extent and scope of nursing work (Bowker & Star, 2000; Sandelowski, 2000). While their linguistic specificity and style of objective reporting present a purely technical event, as the next section shows, the time and space of wound care comprises moments of negotiation, expression of needs and wants, and the flesh and blood realities of tending large wounds that result from burn trauma. What these ethnographic data accomplish in the exploration of nursing practice, as Willis (2000) asserts, is a resistance to the pure abstraction of textual records and the forms of analysis such texts allow.

Nursing and patient desires with/in the social space of 'the dressing'

In the following sections, I describe and analyse two different wound care observations for the ways in which nurse and patient desires surface in the interactions. My use of the term 'desire' is deliberate, although, I recognise, contentious in some respects. However, in current cultural studies techniques, the use of such a term signals the emotional import embedded in wound care practices and has stronger connotations than the use of other concepts such as strategies, agendas or negotiations. Also, the use of the psychoanalytical term 'desire' conveys (analytically) how not all meaning-making is explicit, but rather is implicit (even unconscious) in language use. I show later in this discussion how such hidden messages can be diagnosed by socio-linguistic approaches to language use (see Fairclough, 1992, 1995).

Moreover, my emphasis on taking a psychoanalytic approach is encouraged by Anzieu's (1989) and Kristeva's (1982) explanations that our relationship to skin is set very early in our emotional development. From such a psychoanalytic understanding, skin and its emotional overlays are reanimated, and nurses' focus on the importance of skin integrity (having a complete skin cover) begins to make sense. This analysis is predicated on the known emotional effects that accompany the destabilisation of skin as a boundary which signals what legitimately lies inside and outside of the body, as these are set by socio-cultural norms and rules (Douglas, 1966;

Kristeva, 1982). When skin integrity is ruptured and does not constitute a complete boundary (physically, emotionally or socially), those who are directly affected by this phenomenon experience all of the horror of such a failure; as do those who witness this destabilisation, that is nurses and other health care workers.

Skin is an underdetermined component in much of our emotional lives, as is the emotional meaning of its completeness to us. It is so completely taken for granted as a boundary, that the horror associated with its potential failure is kept at bay by many firmly held psychosocial beliefs. All of the certainties encouraged by these beliefs are swept away when its fabric is ruptured. Also, skin is acknowledged as a major contributor to our human capability of communicating emotions such as intimacy, embarrassment and joy. Skin conveys a sense of our identity through the maintenance of its boundaries (Anzieu, 1989). It remains as a taken-for-granted background until it becomes injured, traumatised or otherwise than normal. In nurses' care for skin, during bathing or wound care procedures, resides much of the intimate work informing nursing knowledge about bodies and bodily practices (Lawler, 1991). In using psychoanalytic concepts to analyse interactions between nurses and patients during wound care procedures, such analysis acknowledges the various forms of relational intimacy which constitute skin and wound care practices, as well as the technical and scientific values that are similarly evident in nursing texts about wounds and wound care (Bland, 1996; Gardner, 1996). However, unlike the standardised formal texts, description and analysis of these interactions discloses how, in each of these occasions, there resides the potential for nurses and patients to work differently because their desires (conscious and unconscious) can drive the care in different and complex directions.

A formative element of nurse and patient identity in this setting results from the way in which their various or similar desires and interests are mobilised in the dressing process itself to re-establish boundaries that are central to our understanding of social identity (Rudge, 1997). Such mobilisation ensures that each interaction between nurse and patient is constituted by a contest over whose desires and interests frame the interactions at any particular moment. As a basis for this analysis, I explore two interactions for the ways in which nurse and patient identity intensifies and produces this social space in terms of body–ego–space (Pile, 1996), where the body and ego are viewed as interacting to produce the emotional meanings that can be mapped and analysed from by a psychoanalytically informed discussion.

Observation one: nursing control meets patient desire

The observation which forms the basis of this analysis is one in which a nurse with long experience in the unit was doing Phil's dressing. This dressing occurred the day after Phil had a painful, traumatic experience when another nurse had done his dressing. He was very nervous about any nurse he could not remember doing his dressing before.

> [Phil had walked down to the bathroom for his shower with Nita and I. Phil was taking off his gown and Nita was organising the chair, the dressing pack which had Phil's dressing requirements in it.]

Phil: I don't seem to be able to bend this bit. Do you think that I'll be able to have the dressing done in my room?

Nita: No, I'll do the dressing here.

Phil: It's just that I get so cold in here ... in the bathroom.

Nita: I'll get the heater put in your bedroom, so it will be warm when you get back. It's easier to do your dressing here.

> [Phil is already shaking. Nita goes out of the room and gets someone to put the heater in Phil's room. She comes back in, puts a plastic apron on, puts on a gown, and plastic gloves. Phil is now standing near the shower with only his dressings on. Nita starts cutting off the surgifix which holds it in place. Phil is lifting his arms out of the way and is *very* quiet for him. Once all of the surgifix is cut off and some of the melolin and 'silvered' chux are taken off, Nita double gloves with sterile gloves and I start the shower. Phil holds the shower head to direct the water over his body and watches as Nita starts taking the dressings off the grafted areas and other parts. She is washing him down with the sponge pad, washing off the cream and exudate from the burnt areas.]

Phil: You have to watch this bit here.

Nita: I know, those bits that have been grafted. I'll make sure that these are soaked before I take them off.

[She deftly removes the paraffin gauze, washes the sections with 'silvers' on them and washes his pubic area to remove the cream and paraffin ointment from the tulle gras.]

Phil: Ah, you're a good one, you're a good one!

[Nita glances at me, and says nothing.]

Phil: Yeah, you're a good one!

Nita: Do you always carry on like this. If you don't stop carrying on, I'll stamp on your foot.

Phil: Don't you want to know? She's a good one!

[This last comment was addressed to me. Nita finishes the shower and dries Phil off with a towel and then moves him into the middle of the room. Phil is supporting himself on the bath. Nita uncovers his dressings, takes off one pair of gloves and starts putting on his dressings. She puts the silvered dressings on the burns, puts previously cut surgifix on to keep this in place and checks the recently grafted areas. Phil is shivering.]

Phil: This white cream is absolutely freezing.

[He is shaking visibly now. Nita quickly finishes the dressing, puts on his new sterile gown and moves Phil back to his room.]

When I talked with Nita after the dressing, I asked her why she had answered Phil in this way. She said that she was embarrassed at the way he was 'carrying on about the dressing' while I was in the room. Other patients at times said these kinds of things to other nurses who were particularly deft with their dressing techniques. Nita was the only one who seemed to be embarrassed by this at the time. Most nurses did not say anything to patients when they said these kinds of things to them. The expected norm for practice in the unit, and one that accompanied expertise and deftness with dressing techniques, was that the nurse would not cause pain during the dressing. Some of this was achieved by the giving of medication at a time which would ensure maximum cover for pain, and when the patient had intravenous lines in place, by the giving of a bolus of medication to cover those moments where there could be extreme pain. Thus a 'good' nurse in this unit would have been someone like Nita – who regularly achieved such an outcome from her dressing technique, with deft, knowledgeable and assured technique.

At the other side of this dressing, is the nurse who did the dressing yesterday, who is by imputation a 'bad' nurse, and who did not achieve the expected normal outcome. However, this recent experience is not mentioned, but is silent background to the entire procedure. On the morning of this dressing there was considerable discussion in the unit over the previous day's experience for Phil, and much discussion on how to avoid these kinds of incident in the future. It had been established that there had been a failure to hand over accurately where there was no record of an area of debrided wound which was covered by tulle gras rather than by donor skin, with the resultant trauma when the tulle was removed at dressing time. Assigning Phil to Nita was a direct result of this previous day's outcome and an attempt to ensure that Phil regained his confidence in the nurses that he had lost yesterday. Therefore, in this case, Nita was dealing with a very nervous patient whom I had observed at other times struggling with nurses, fighting with them over control of the sponge or the razor and very loud and abusive in his combat. On this occasion, while he did try to negotiate a more comfortable location for his re-dressing, he surrendered to the nurse's ability to do his dressing without 'hurting' him. Such a surrender exemplifies how the patient's understandable desire not to be hurt meets with nursing expertise to bring about a specific form of patient interaction with nurses: the 'thankful' patient.

Also, the above observation exposes how some nurses positioned themselves (and the patients) during the dressing process. The nurse in this case is driving how the dressing occurs, as well as the pace of the dressing. What allows this is her ability and her 'technical' expertise with dressings. The whole dressing was done very quickly with very little interaction between patient and nurse, even when some comment is asked for by the patient. In her comment that it is easier to do the dressing in the bathroom, much is hidden from the patient in such a statement. For instance, the bathroom allowed ease of access to the standing patient's body rather than the bedroom which was crowded with equipment, making the dressing easier to complete. Also, going back to the room before completion of the dressing exposes the patient's uncovered wounds to the potential of cross-infection in the 'unclean' corridor. The nurse does not mention that the dressings themselves will make him cold as they are infiltrated with a cold cream that will be cold no matter where the dressing occurs. Under the cover of 'ease' of dressing are many unexplained matters, unexplained to the patient at this time, or as part of her explanation to me after the dressing is complete.

Observation two: unconscious nursing desire meets patient desire

The observation which forms the basis of this section is one where Brett is having his dressing done by Ken. Brett has just had grafting done to his arms and yet is still needing to have burnt areas on his abdomen washed while he is in bed and these dressings replaced. This excerpt of the entire observation is where Ken was washing and changing the 'silver' on Brett's burnt areas of skin. Ken is assisted by a junior nurse, who is actually responsible for the rest of Brett's care. Ken is doing the dressing because graft care has been done, and the other nurse has no experience with this aspect of care. At this stage, Brett is still having to have his grafted arms splinted to prevent movement, and then raised on a system of pulleys. This means that he cannot use his arms and hands to move around the bed, or to stabilise himself, or importantly, to reposition his dressings on his still burnt stomach. As these dressings have silver sulphadiazine on them they are slippery and this is compounded by the continuous loss of exudate from under the full thickness burns.

Ken: Now how have you been managing with these dressings?
Brett: Well I have been noticing that by the end of the day, these ones on my body here [pointing to stomach]. They seem to slip up and then drip everywhere.
Ken: OK. I can manage to do that better. I will make sure that I tie the surgifix up so that it doesn't slip. Is there any parts in particular, that you find uncomfortable? Any sore parts?
Brett: What apart from the donor part?

Ken: Mm. Any parts that I should be a bit careful with. Does it hurt when the dressing slips up?

Brett: Yeah, that part is really sore.

Ken: Yeah, looks a bit red around the bottom [lifting sheet off the lower body to look at the bottom of the burnt area]. Well, we'll try and fix that.

[Ken begins washing the burnt area with saline and a clean chux. The other male nurse assists by putting more warm saline in the bowl when Brett says it's a bit cold. Ken works quickly, cleaning, and then placing the new silvered dressings in place. He then spends a great deal of time (timed at 7 minutes) getting Brett to move around in the bed to put the surgifix on the dressings, tying them to the arms, to the dressings on the legs so that the surgifix is securely kept down.]

Ken: How's that? Does that feel OK? After all we can't have that slipping up can we, after I've said it won't? [laughs and Brett laughs with him] Now it's really important to me that you are comfortable with this.

Brett: Yeah, it's great. At least we don't have to worry about my arms bending at the moment.

Ken: Yeah, they have to keep still because of the grafts, remember. We can help with anything you need to use your arms for. [One of Brett's arms is in a splint, and one is raised by a pulley system.] Now remember, to keep them still won't you? [Brett nods.]

[Ken and the junior nurse change his bed linen. Brett has to roll from side to side and is moved up the bed. This takes a further 10 minutes to get him 'right' as they have to replace the bed foam and bottom sheet, and dispose of the bed foam into a plastic bag and the sheets soiled with blood and exudate mixed with 'silvers' into the linen skip. When this is complete Ken asks:]

Ken: Now, now are those dressings still in place? [Brett nods and grins.]

Brett: They better had after all the time you spent on them.

Ken: Absolutely! My reputation is resting on it. Still it's really important that *you* are comfortable with it. It's really important to me that you are.

[Ken and the junior nurse clean up the room. The dressing procedure has taken 90 minutes, at least 30 minutes of this on the dressings to the burnt areas still remaining on Brett's body.]

As I came out of the room for the dressing, another senior nurse is coming out of another patient's room. She makes a comment about Ken taking twice as long as anyone else to do a dressing. This is obvious also when a comparison is made between Observation One which took 20 minutes and the time taken by Ken (90 minutes). In fact, this was a common aspect of Ken's practice. He told me during his final interview that he considers the time taken during the dressing to discuss issues with the patient is a very important part of the 'counselling' aspects of the nursing role in the unit.

However, analysis of this interaction and others I have recorded, indicates that Ken's interactions were largely didactic and instrumental, rather than interactions which dealt with emotional issues for the patient. May (1990), in an extensive review of research into nurse–patient interactions, characterises such interactions as technocratic and instrumental, rather than relational. Moreover, this is a space and time which is largely imbued with nursing desire: the desire for patient comfort as an estimation of nursing worth. As such, this particular space is as controlled by nursing issues as by those of the patient. What the nurse indicates too, is that patient comfort and staying comfortable was important 'to me'. Moreover, this aspect is in concordance with the patients' desire.

Ken was very skilled with the dressing procedures in the unit. He had been working in the unit for just over ten years and this was evident in his ability to deal with most kinds of dressing and techniques. He was also skilful in diverting the patient and keeping them amused with a constant flow of jokes, patter, and talk about the dressing, the wound and the various technologies needed to care for the skin. However, such a constant patter did not allow much 'space' for differing kinds of relational work. The patients, moreover, were more often than not happy to leave the interaction at that level. Thus Ken created a space, where like Nita, the patients felt safe 'under' his hands. Such a focus on expertise with their skin also enabled patients to achieve some control over the technical aspects of wound care highly valued within the forces for self-care in the unit.

Moreover, this was a key component of the patients achieving some sense of 'certainty'. In building this space, within the dressing procedure itself, Ken also made sure, like other nurses, that the information he provided was immediately relevant to the patient and their phase of recovery. On one level, interactions such as these in wound care procedures meet the conscious 'desires' of nursing work. They also are evidence of many of the 'unconscious' desires which colour some nursing interactions. My 'sense' of this form of nurse–patient interaction is that it is evoked by the 'unconscious' need for affirmation of a particular nurse's worth. While Nita met such approval and acclaim from the patient with 'diffidence' and refusal (because of my presence?), Ken was seeking some 'unconscious' rewards of such talented work.

The social space of wound care practices

In this final section I discuss aspects of the preceding analysis. In particular, I focus on the variations in practices, rather than their standardisation. This firstly will be through an examination of the movement between the various forms of care. I follow this with a discussion of how this space is invested with competing and complementary desires of nurses and patients, emphasising the intersections and gaps between the way nurses and patients constitute this spatio-temporal event.

Working with and on bodies: spatial practices

As has been suggested throughout this chapter, nurses worked in a variety of ways with the implements and accoutrements of wound care procedures. In the nurses' discussions of this work, they emphasised how learning had been a 'hands-on' process, where they had learnt from 'doing' the dressing, with a more experienced nurse providing the 'practised' eye for the wound healing process itself. In exploring these notions of skin, dressings as covering, and descriptions of actions during dressings illuminate this mundane practice. This analysis is predicated on the understanding that the body, in nursing, is one of its constant spatial elements (Lawler, 1991; Parker, 1997; Rudge, 1998); just as an architect would consider bricks and mortar the material for building or constructing their particular spatial artefacts.

As I highlighted in the earlier discussion of the wound care observations, there is movement to and fro, between the technological imperatives of the dressing, the negotiations between nurses and patients, the emotional content of pain and its effect, and moments of interaction which could be termed 'therapeutic'. Such observations begin to discern the 'richness' of nurses' and patients' interactions which are never fully captured in the official texts of nursing reports or care plans. In taking this approach, I contend also that this opens up for exploration the variations in nursing practices that so frequently lead nurses to reject these 'texts' as incapable of conveying the complexity of their practice (Bowker and Star, 2000). Through the use of ideas about social space, the contradictions in nursing's regulatory practices around account- ability and documentation are exposed as well. It is not just that nurses' work is not *in* a textbook, but also that its complexity and richness are impossible to capture in such a genre. For this reason, procedure manuals, care plans and patient notes are merely repre- sentations of nursing space–time. However, it is this very impossi- bility that leads nursing to be, as Sandelowski (2000) puts this, the glue in health care system, whose very invisibility enables the organisational work to be accomplished (Latimer, 1998). Also it is important to recognise that such textual representations are ideo- logical in their effects.

As I indicated in the beginning section of this chapter, the 'offi- cial' texts of wound care, that is the care plans and nursing notes, are comparatively empty. This emptiness is more apparent when compared with the two observations of practice which inform this chapter. Such an effect is compounded by nurses routinising their notes to very simplistic or cursory representations in the case notes such as 'Dressings ✓'. These notes equally constitute the patient as 'absent' except as a wound or dressing. This absence, as other authors have noted (Parker & Gardner, 1992; Cheek & Rudge, 1994; Latimer, 1997), results from the objective reporting style of notes. I suggest that such a process emerges from the 'standardised' style of care plans (Timmermans *et al.*,

1998). Moreover, this form of analysis suggests that a focus on 'texts' alone would provide only a partial record of such a nursing event, leaving the analysis open to critiques similar to those Lefebvre (1991) levels against 'pure' textual research. Indeed, he argues that analysis of spatial practices re-peoples discourse analytic studies. I believe it also endows such analysis with the 'real' effects of these texts on the people who inhabit such spaces (McRobbie, 1997; Willis, 2000).

As indicated in the observations of practice, nurses' practice towards the body, with their bodies and with the implements of wound care are various. Such practices can be attending to the dressings, washing the wounds, re-covering with dressings and bandages and teaching the patient about their wound care. As such these practices indicate how nurses' embodied practices towards and with the patients' bodies are as variable as the requirements of each dressing and its social space. For these reasons, the ordering of relations through care plans, procedure manuals or written documentation forms a 'rhetorical space' (Code, 1995) where such regulations adopt standardised expressions about nurse–patient relationships and form a mere background to the personal and situational expression of nurse–patient interactions evidenced in observational data.

As Bowker & Star (2000) suggest, classificatory systems and information management systems such as medical records, nursing care plans and in-record checks all conspire in the process of organisational forgetting and erasure of nursing work. I would also add that they promote a forgetting that counts much more widely than the organisations themselves. However, nurses and patients in their everyday interactions know and recognise, as one nurse put this, 'that it is nurses' work which walks out of the unit on the patients' bodies'. While this analysis indicates how nursing space is inhabited by and imbued with the dominant concerns of medical technology, it is also informed by cultural understandings concerning the body and bodily functions in health and illness as well as the body's corporeal presence (Lupton, 1994). It is these variabilities that are difficult to convey in all of nursing's official records (organisational and professional), and continue to provide nurses with methods to refuse such ideologically driven imperatives – a position not without its rewards or dangers.

Complementary and contradictory desires in a social space

In these considerations of the professional and personal coordinates that intersect in the social space of the dressing, I believe the desires invested in such a space have both conscious and unconscious effects (Lefebvre, 1991; Pile, 1996). In particular, these effects relate to the way in which taboos and rules of exclusion and inclusion interact with the chaotic and 'braided' horrors of the wounded body (Kristeva, 1982). The threats presented by the wounded body constantly challenge ideologies and knowledge systems set up to control for its effects. Indeed, as Kristeva's analysis of abjection (an emotional defence) suggests, the very presence of such rules acknowledges the constancy of abjection as *always already* present whenever boundaries are destabilised. Hence, I emphasise the centrality of desire in the operations that underpin the will to cover, control or acknowledge abjection, as part of all wound care processes (Rudge, 1998) and as evident within spoken texts and practices of nurses and patients. Further, the notion of 'desire' allows an account of the way that this space is produced as both a conscious and 'unconscious' reality.

Even the desire for erasure present in the emotionally impoverished official accounts can be read as a form of continued resistance to the things that bureaucracies consider to 'count'. By the continuation of such acts of erasure, nurses continue to keep secret the talented and accomplished work they do to 'glue' the system together (Sandelowski, 2000). Similarly, nursing texts, consciously or unconsciously, are attempts by nurses to control the emotionality of the spaces of wound care. Such a process is also evident in the way in which nurses control the processes of wound care, and set the tempo of each dressing. Also, nursing desire is evident in competent practice, technical skill and the outcome of patient comfort. Patient desires are discernible in the way that they negotiate for their own comfort, surrender to nursing expertise, or work to obtain some control over their skin or pain management. Also in these interactions, there is evidence that patients undertake a dualistic categorisation of nursing practice into good or bad nursing. This is done according to the parameters of their classificatory system, where measures such as control over pain, expertise and the nurses' willingness to allow some negotiation are some of the indicators.

I assert that the desire to cover and dress seek to control the abject wounded body while simultaneously intensifying the relations of power/knowledge embedded in this nursing procedure. These desires colour the space–time in which the nurses work with the patients. The practices embedded in these encounters between nurses and patients with their textual influences, their embodied selves and the representations that governed these, come together in the creation of a social space: 'the dressing'. Self-evidently, this space is a social space, as well as one where the structural effects on nurses' (and less recognisably, patients') are apparent.

Moreover, systems of meaning, nurse and patient identity and representations of nursing and patienthood leak into and colour this space (Kristeva, 1982; Pile, 1996; Bauman, 2001). Despite the constraints set by organisational acts of erasure, the space of 'the dressing' (or indeed any act of bodily intimacy) always has the potential to be taken over by 'transgressive' emotions. These emotions are, nevertheless, often apprehended unconsciously and 'protected' from exposure by the barriers put up against their intrusion into the process. For instance, Ken, on one level in his interaction with Brett, is giving the impression, legitimate in much of the nursing literature on caring, that the patient's comfort is *first*. However, in his use of pronouns (see Fairclough, 1995) in his iterative statements – 'Now its really important to *me* that *you* are comfortable with this' – and his reiteration of this at the completion of the dressing: 'Absolutely! *My* reputation is resting on it. Still it's really important that *you* are comfortable with it. It's really important to *me* that *you* are [comfortable]', he is unconsciously signalling transgressive emotions often unrecognised in formalised nursing texts. In locating himself first in this sentence, Ken is suggesting 'unconsciously' that it is me (and hence, my reputation and motivation) that is central in his practice.

While Fox (1994), following Cixous (1996), would suggest that this is a gift, an endowment to patients, I would suggest that such pleasures and desires are what keeps nurses such as Nita and Ken doing what they do for their many years of practice in this unit. Such pleasure resides at the other side of 'horror' and makes such longevity of tenure understandable at an emotional level. Moreover, while these pleasures are difficult to account for if one looks at the 'horror' of a burn trauma, it explains how nurses continue to work in such areas. In covering the horror with the pleasure derived from such accomplished practice, nurses recognise and acknowledge such horror while controlling for its presence in their working lives. Not to do so would make such work difficult to bear. Paradoxically, and more importantly, such recognition constantly works against the space of erasure in which nursing is located and this emotional space may have some relevance in retaining experienced nurses to work in such challenging areas. Nurses and the patients (under their hands) know that 'it' (pleasure) counts and makes a difference in the everyday world of these nursing practices.

Methodological considerations

Research which surfaces such complexity (and of course, its dissemination) participates in another form of 'unforgetting' that is as significant as the developers of nursing informatics systems, writing nursing into hospital records and the other endless calls to document 'nursing'. It is writing with political intent. Bowker & Star (2000) note that the developers of one such nursing documentation system (Nursing Intervention Classification, NIC) sought to rewrite nursing without its history. Pre-NIC was determined as unscientific, a-theoretical and worse still, unable to be substantiated. My argument throughout this chapter has been that words are indeed powerful tools, to influence and shape how nursing practice is conceptualised as well as ways of describing and analysing nursing practice. As a witness to such practices and a recorder of nursing in text, and through its texts, I am advocating an ethnographic attitude towards nursing practice (Haraway, 1997) that emphasises context, history and the unsubstantiated as important in nursing practice. I assume that there is much that requires to be made visible through an active questioning of the web of texts that intersect through and across nursing practices such as wound care.

Further, I want to advocate for nurses using qualitative methodologies to develop and use an ethnographic imagination (Willis, 2000) which encourages an eclectic use of concepts to illuminate the everyday world of nursing practice. Willis suggests such a use of explanatory theories makes explicit the meaning making in the context of any practice world. Concomitantly, this use of theoretical concepts, of necessity, should expose how structural forces operate in practice settings, and are reproduced or resisted 'in practice'. Therefore in this study, the local languages and knowledges that guide and shape practice are analysed, through an application of discourse analytic methods, to identify discourses and their ideological effects as these influence, obfuscate or interrupt the everyday world of nursing practice.

Against a background of the collection of a Foucauldian 'archive' (Foucault, 1972), I have sought to make visible the multiple voices and effects that exist simultaneously within a singular representation of nursing practice (see Bowker & Star, 2000) – the dressing of large wounds resulting from extensive burn trauma. In such a setting, through an analysis of the social actions, the localised agency of the nurses and patients, I have employed an array of theories and concepts, including the psychoanalytic concept of desire, the theories of post-structuralism as these relate to language use, sociolinguistics, and concepts from social space formation to present this complexity, always with the understanding that many other stories could be told from this data.

Conclusion

In this chapter, I outlined the use of qualitative, ethnographic research to explore a circumscribed area of nursing practice – wound care in a burns unit. Such an analysis is informed by the need to explore how the various technologies intersect and interact to produce the wound care procedure as a spatio-temporal event. This event contains within it the interactions between nurses and patients at a moment of great vulnerability and intimacy. The official texts describing this work to (re)cover a person with extensive burn trauma are only one side of the story, one that is standardised to capture aspects that count to the health care system. These elements are not always the 'things' that nurses and patients themselves think matter.

Throughout the event itself, nurses and patients are subjected to the powerful influences of scientific and relational discourses, they took particular subject positions, and participated in an ordering of knowledge(s) about wounds and their care as these occur in the rhetorical space of the 'daily dressing'. As a particular form of time and location, wound care procedures show the effects of dominant discursive framing by science, nursing belief systems and other socio-cultural beliefs. At times, its inhabitants are governed by the way in which this space is 'sterilised' of its corporeality: flesh, blood and power (Moore, 1988). As shown throughout this chapter, elements which are real, symbolic and invested with imaginary power (desire) are implicated in the talk and practices. Moreover, following Pile (1996), I assert that 'space', as a representation, is socially and emotionally constituted 'by maps of meaning and power' (Pile, 1996: 209). As Pile suggests too, this analysis is informed by understandings which assert that the body is a space. A space moreover, which has:

> 'simultaneously real, imagined and symbolic spatialities, which are (all) constituted through experiencing of the social body. Once again, bodies are maps of meaning and power, but where these maps subsist in multiple dimensions of space and time.' (Pile, 1996: 209)

In describing the differences in nurses' and patients' approaches to this singular event, it can be seen that strength may well lie in variety not standardisation. While hegemonic discursive frames shape nurse and patient interactions, contestations and contradictions surface in the shape each interaction takes. Nurses and patients therefore position themselves 'dynamically' within this very static moment of the dressing. Analysis of these dynamics suggests how nurses' and patients' space and time is consumed and produced in such movement and stasis (Lefebvre, 1991). The way in which 'nursing' and nurses (and patients) are best represented is not by recourse to simplistic ideological positions, but by an attempt to convey how such a process is imbued with the multiple realities of human action and speech. Moreover, it is obvious that nursing practice takes place in representational space and time, or lived social space, where nurse researchers confront and are challenged by what does, or does not occur, according to various ideologies of nursing. This is so because nursing practice, so located, is co-opted by, and also resistant to many of nursing's key ideological imperatives as well as to rules and ordering such ideologies seek to impose.

References

Anzieu, D. (1989) *The Skin Ego*. (C. Turner, trans.), New Haven, CT: Yale University Press.

Bauman, Z. (2001) *The Individualized Society*. Cambridge: Polity Press.

Bland, M. (1996) More than just a bit of a nark: living with chronic leg ulcers. *Primary Intention: The Australian Journal of Wound Management* **4** (4): 17–19.

Bowker, G. & Star, S.L. (2000) *Sorting Things Out: Classification and Its Consequences*. Cambridge, MA: MIT Press.

Burman, E. & Parker, I. (eds) (1993) *Discourse Analytic Research: Repertoires and Readings of Text in Action*. London: Routledge.

Cheek, J. & Rudge, T. (1994) Webs of documentation: the discourse of case notes. *Australian Journal of Communication* **13**: 41–52.

Cixous, H. (1996) Sorties. In H. Cixous & C. Clement (eds) *The Newly Born Woman* (B. Wing, trans.). London: I.B. Tauris, pp. 63–132.

Code, L. (1995) *Rhetorical Spaces: Essays on Gendered Locations*. New York: Routledge.

Douglas, M. (1966) *Purity and Danger*. London: Routledge & Kegan Paul.

Fairclough, N. (1992) *Discourse and Social Change*. Cambridge: Polity Press.

Fairclough, N. (1995) *Media Discourses*. London: Routledge.

Foucault, M. (1970) *The Order of Things* (unidentified collective translation). London: Tavistock.

Foucault, M. (1972) *The Archeology of Knowledge* (A.M. Sheridan, trans.). London: Tavistock.

Fox, N. (1994) *Postmodernism, Sociology and Health*. Toronto: University of Toronto Press.

Gardner, G. (1996) The walking wounded. *Primary Intention: The Australian Journal of Wound Management* **4** (4): 5–8.

Haraway, D. (1997) *Feminism and Technoscience:* Modest-Witness@ Second_MilleniumFemaleMan©_Meets_OncoMouse™. New York: Routledge.

Kristeva, J. (1982) *Powers of Horror: An Essay on Abjection* (L.S. Roudiez, trans.). New York: Columbia University Press.

Latimer, J. (1997) Giving patients a future: the constitution of classes in an acute medical unit. *Sociology of Health and Illness* **19**: 160–85.

Latimer, J. (1998) Organizing context: nurses' assessments of older people in an acute medical unit. *Nursing Inquiry* **5**: 43–57.

Lawler, J. (1991) *Behind the Screens: Nursing, Somology, and the Problem of the Body*. Melbourne: Churchill Livingstone.

Lefebvre, H. (1991) *The Production of Space* (D. Nicholson-Smith, trans.). Oxford: Blackwell.

Lupton, D. (1994) *Medicine as Culture: Illness, Disease and the Body in Western Societies*. London: Sage.

May, C. (1990) Research on nurse–patient relationships: problems of theory, problems of practice. *Journal of Advanced Nursing* **15**: 307–15.

May, C. (1992) Nursing work, nurse's knowledge, and the subjectification of the patient. *Sociology of Health and Illness* **13**: 472–87.

McRobbie, A. (1997) *More!* New sexualities in girls' and women's magazines. In A. McRobbie (ed.) *Back to Reality? Social Experience and Cultural Studies*. Manchester: Manchester University Press, pp. 190–209.

Moore, S. (1988) Getting a bit of the other – the pimps of postmodernism. In R. Chapman & J. Rutherford, (eds) *Male Order: unwrapping masculinity*. London: Lawrence & Wishart, pp. 165–92.

Parker, J. (1997) The body as text and the body as living flesh: metaphors of the body and nursing postmodernity. In J. Lawler (ed.) *The Body in Nursing: A Collection of Views*. Melbourne: Churchill Livingstone, pp. 11–29.

Parker, J. & Gardner, G. (1992) The silence and the silencing of the nurse's voice: a reading of patient progress notes. *Australian Journal of Advanced Nursing* **9** (2): 3–9.

Pile, S. (1996) *The Body and the City: Psychoanalysis, Space and Subjectivity*. London: Routledge.

Rudge, T. (1997) *Nursing wounds: a discourse analysis of interactions between nurses and patients during wound care procedures in a burns unit*. PhD dissertation, La Trobe University, Melbourne, Australia.

Rudge, T. (1998) Skin as cover: the discursive effects of 'covering' metaphors on wound care practices. *Nursing Inquiry* **5**: 228–37.

Rudge, T. (1999) Situating wound management: technoscience, dressings and 'other' skins. *Nursing Inquiry* **6**: 167–77.

Sandelowski, M. (2000) *Devices and Desires: Gender, Technology and American Nursing*. Chapel Hill: University of North Carolina Press.

Silverman, D. (1993) *Interpreting Qualitative Data: Methods for Analysing Talk, Text and Interaction*. London: Sage.

Timmermanns, S., Bowker, G.C. & Star, S.L. (1998) The architecture of difference: visibility, control and comparability in building a nursing interventions classification. In M. Berg & A. Mol (eds) *Difference in Medicine: Unraveling Practices, Techniques, and Bodies*. Durham, NC: Duke University Press, pp. 202–225.

Wicks, D. (1999) *Nurses and Doctors at Work: Rethinking Professional Boundaries*. St Leonards, NSW: Allen & Unwin.

Willis, P. (2000) *The Ethnographic Imagination*. Oxford: Polity Press.

PART V

Materials

Many of the preceding authors help us to realise that nursing practice and patienthood is much more than just physical. But they also insist on the materiality of patienthood and of nursing. Bodies, machines, thermometers, dressings, charts and records are just some of the materials and technologies which nurses engage with in their day-to-day practice. 'Things', however, are never just functional: the meanings materials have go way beyond their practical use (as, for example, tools) or the talk that displays them.

That materials are 'symbols of significance' is well rehearsed in the anthropological literature. These kinds of materials include

> 'words for the most part but also gestures, drawings, musical sounds, mechanical devices like clocks, or natural objects like jewels – anything in fact that is disengaged from its mere actuality and used to impose meaning upon experience.' (Geertz, 1993: 45)

From an anthropological perspective, *significance* is substantiated, in words and other cultural materials. By attending 'to the world of goods', and to the practices around them, we can offer distinct understandings of how the social is made up (Douglas and Isherwood, 1980). The chapters in Part V focus on the materiality of nursing, and present approaches to interpretation which illuminate nurses' identity-work as well as the socio-political and cultural context which nurses' work helps to reproduce.

References

Douglas, M. and Baron Isherwood (1980) *The World of Goods: Towards an Anthropology of Consumption*. Harmondsworth: Penguin.

Geertz, C. (1993) *The Interpretation of Cultures*. London: Fontana.

CHAPTER 10

Taking things seriously: studying the material culture of nursing

Margarete Sandelowski

A hitherto neglected focus of qualitative nursing inquiry has been the physical objects comprising the material world and culture of nursing. All kinds of things, from beds to computers, populate and shape the world of the nurse. These things have been described – like people – as having agency, biographies, histories, idiosyncratic quirks, and 'known propensities for perverse or benign behavior' (Callon, 1995; Orr, 1996: 89; Prout, 1996; Wiener *et al.*, 1997). These things not only help nurses care for their patients, but also 'embody [nurses'] goals, make [their] skills manifest, and shape [their] identities' (Csikszentmihalyi & Rochberg-Halton, 1981: 1). As makers and users of objects, human beings are also reflections of the things they make and use.

Qualitative researchers have tended to favor verbal over non-verbal sources of data: that is, interviews over observations, documents and artefacts (Silverman, 1998). As Atkinson & Silverman (1997) proposed, interviews, while giving voice to persons often unheard in society, may also give us a false sense of authentic experience. Yet in the study of the things people use, covet, fear, and reject lies the opportunity to offset the politically correct tendency to accept interview data as the best reflection of the private self and another means 'to understand what people are and what they might become' (Csikszentmihalyi & Rochberg-Halton, 1981: 1). In the study of the material culture of a group lies a means to get closer to the lived and storied experiences qualitative researchers strive to re-present faithfully, especially those of cultures, like nursing, with strong non-verbal traditions and practices.

Accordingly, in this chapter, I address issues related to and approaches for the study of things, and the significance of this focus of inquiry for nursing. I define things here as physical objects[1] having weight and mass and available, accessible, and belonging to both the eye and the hand. I draw from scholarship in material culture studies; social science, cultural and gender studies of technology; and, in the history of technology, especially medical and nursing technology.

Learning from things

Scholars have typically not taken physical objects as seriously as they might or should (Corn, 1996: 35). Like other scholars in fields where things have primacy, nurses have tended to emphasize knowing about things, as opposed to knowing or 'learning (directly) from things' (Kingery, 1996). Although they learn, and teach each other, how to use things (for example, how to give an injection, how to change a dressing, how to read an EKG strip), nurses have yet to study the things at hand's end as extensions of their hands, or as artefacts of culture and history. They have yet to draw evidence about practice from their 'firsthand encounter(s)' (Corn, 1996: 44) with the 'thingness' (p. 43) of things.

There are several reasons for this lack of attention in the practice and social science disciplines. First (and as I discuss in more detail later), things are not easy to interpret and they, therefore, may not be the best sources of evidence, even in studies directly concerned with things (Lawrence, 1992; Corn, 1996).

The privileging of mind over matter

Second, there has been a long-standing western (North American and western European) cultural tendency of privileging mind over matter, and the brain over the hand: that is, of favoring the cerebral and abstract over the manual, material and concrete. Indeed, the concept of 'material culture' contains its own contradiction as westerners associate the word 'material' with the base and pragmatic and the word 'culture' with the lofty and intellectual (Prown, 1996). Graduate education, in particular, contributes to the primacy of the 'cognitive, the theorized, and the abstract over the experiential, the ordinary, and the personally particularised', as 'tactile, visual, or experiential' accounts are more likely to be considered 'personal' than 'professional' or scholarly. 'Being "objective" paradoxically may require suppressing experience with actual objects' (Corn, 1996: 46–7).

Not only has there been a western intellectual antipathy to the material in favor of the mental, but a denial of the mental in the material. Ferguson (1977: 835) argued that the 'nonliterary and nonscientific … intellectual component of technology', the origins of which lie in art, has been increasingly de-emphasized with the growing influence of science. Yet, 'nonverbal knowledge' plays the crucial part in decisions concerning the 'form, arrangement, and texture' of objects (p. 835). The study of things offers an entrée to knowledge that cannot be expressed in language. Especially relevant to nursing, the knowledge contained in 'material practice' involves 'implicit taken-for-granted skill or know-how' (Hodder, 2000: 708).

Moreover, such study can offset the limitations of language. Kouwenhoven (1982) was concerned that scholars tend to accept verbal evidence as if it were equivalent to sensory evidence. Contrasting the 'generalizing characteristic' (p. 83) of words with the particulars of experience, he argued that the word 'grass' suggests an identity between blades of grass that are in actuality not wholly like each other. This 'suggestion of identity encourages us to disregard the different looks, feels, tastes, and smells of the uncounted blades that comprise the actuality of grass as we experience it' (p. 83). Accordingly, two people talking about grass can be in 'verbal agreement' (both using 'grass' to refer ostensibly to the same thing), without necessarily 'meaning the same thing' (p. 83). They are 'interpret[ing] reality by words, instead of interpreting words by the specific realities of which they are symbols' (p. 84). They share a western cultural 'weakness for mistaking words for things' (p. 86). For Kouwenhoven, verbal evidence is not enough to know culture, not only because of the 'radical limitations of words' (p. 83), but also because many people do not speak for themselves: or, as in the case of nurses, use other non-verbal means of communication and expression, or have been silenced. For Kouwenhoven, who emphasized the limitations of words in order to 'remove the chief obstacle to the consideration of things … American culture is expressed more adequately in the Brooklyn Bridge than in the poem

Hart Crane wrote about it' (p. 87). Trachtenberg's study of the Brooklyn Bridge (1979) demonstrates well how a bridge can 'articulate in objective form the important ideas and feelings of [a] culture' (p. ix).

In the history and culture of western nursing, the hand, and the things at hand's end, have been seen to handicap nurses: that is, to divert them from their efforts to represent nursing as an intellectual practice (Sandelowski, 2000). Nurses seeking to secure the place of nursing in the academy have worked to construct 'the mind of nursing' (Hamilton, 1994), and to theorize and 'etherealize' (Dunlop, 1986: 664) it, in order to flee the handmaiden and physician's-hand image of nursing. Disembodying and dematerializing nursing, they have located it beyond the hand and body work – or the embodied practices – that distinguish it from other professions (Lawler, 1991). Adhering to western cultural hierarchies that rank mind over matter and brain over hand, nurses have thus inadvertently undermined their own culture and overlooked an important source of evidence about it.

The denial of the material in the material

A third reason for the lack of attention to things lies in the emergence of a distinctively postmodern world view whereby matter is conceived as no longer necessarily material. While the modern tendency has been to deny the mental in the material, the postmodern tendency has been to deny the *material* in the material. For example, technology studies scholars who view technologies as socially constructed and/or gender-coded have sought to avoid charges of technological determinism (a view of technology as a key driving force for change) by denying the primacy of physical objects in their conceptualizations of technology. Eager to escape the 'tyranny of things' (Oldenziel, 1996: 58), these scholars argue for a view of technology as a socio/cultural configuration of people, purposes, knowledge, and things in which things play only a minor role. They emphasize the interpretative, as opposed to material (as, for example, in plastic and rubber), flexibility of technology (Bijker *et al.*, 1987).

Indeed, turn-of-the-twenty-first-century information technology does call into question the materiality of things, as it entails a virtual reality neither accessible to direct sensation nor comprehensible by commonsense notions of space and time (Hine, 2000). As Alexandra Chasin (1995: 75) observed: the 'materiality of electronic machines is so elusive . . . it's as though there's no there there'. Yet there is still a materiality to this technology – its hardware and software – that cannot be denied and without which *immaterial* information could not be produced. Moreover, as Hayles (1993: 149) noted, this technology is reconfiguring our very bodies (also depicted in post-modern discourses as immaterial and even irrelevant) by altering our 'habits of posture, eye focus, hand motions, and neural connections'. For example, the touch required to produce text on a computer keyboard is lighter than on a manual typewriter. With the type-writer, the heavier the touch, the darker the text produced; with the computer keyboard, the weight of touch makes no difference to the shade of the text. In addition, as Hayles (1993: 165) described it:

> 'The material resistance of the text to manipulation has dramatically decreased. To erase an error on a manually typed page, it was necessary to interact physically with the paper. Touch was heavy – my fingers used to ache after pounding away on my old Smith-Corona for a couple of hours – and the resistance of materiality was immediately and physically present.'

In nursing practice, the materiality of the computerized patient record is dramatically altering the information behavior and body 'habits' (Hayles, 1993: 157) of nurses by requiring very different eye and hand movements and perceptual skills than the paper record. By virtue of its weight and mass, the paper record can be held or might even be too heavy or too bulky to manage with one hand. With the computer record, there appears to be 'no there there' as it has no physical presence, except 'in there' on screen and 'out there' in cyberspace. Although postmodern ideas and tech-nologies have called into question the lines westerners have typi-cally drawn between human and not-human, mind and body, and mental and material, there is still a materiality even to virtual things that is hardly immaterial to our understanding of changes in human behavior and even physical capabilities. The human body is more than an 'immaterial informational structure . . . [whose] being . . . is concentrated in the brain and the genetic code' (Hayles, 1993: 148).

While the objects nurses use have a 'social presence through their participation in [a] social world', they also have an 'irreducible core' as physical entities (Orr, 1996: 3) with physical effects.

Material culture studies

'Material culture' can be defined as encompassing 'the totality of artifacts in a culture, the vast universe of objects used by human-kind to cope with the physical world, to facilitate social intercourse, to delight our fancy, and to create symbols of meaning' (Schlereth, 1982: 2), including objects as diverse as written texts, ritual symbols, and roads. Human-made or human-modified 'physical objects are crucial to what constitutes material culture' (p. 2). A 'natural object' such as a stone becomes a 'material object', or a 'physical manifestation of culture' (p. 2), when someone uses or alters it for some purpose, such as jewelry or warfare.

The material culture of nursing includes such three-dimensional health care devices, often referred to as tools, instruments, and/or technologies, as thermometers, therapeutic beds, infusion pumps and monitors, and such everyday objects as telephones and toilets. Also included are such three-dimensional written documents as textbooks, the paper patient record, patient education brochures, and procedure manuals and the two-dimensional texts they contain. The material culture of nursing also includes the visual products of objects such as computers and monitors, including rhythm strips, sonographic and X-ray images, printouts, graphic and numeric displays, charts, tables, drawings and photos. These visual products comprise the media of clinical practice, which is increasingly mediated by them (Sandelowski, 1998, 2001). Indeed, amongst the most dramatic features of western health care at the turn of the twenty-first century is the increasing turn to and triumph of 'phantasmic images' (Stafford, 1994: 281) of animated fetuses, beating hearts and other internal organs once hidden from view. Scientific practices of all kinds now largely comprise these images and 'inscriptions' (Latour & Woolgar, 1986), which make objects visible and 'analyzable' as scientific data (Lynch, 1985: 37). For example, photographs have played a critical role in the history of medicine, in general, and in the 'icnonographies of wound care', in particular, documenting but also re-presenting patients, health and disease (Rudge, 1999: 171). Our concept of human anatomy almost wholly comprises of anatomical drawings that construct, rather than simply portray, the human body (Moore & Clarke, 1995). Anatomical knowledge is 'medium dependent' (Waldby, 2000: 90), changing when the medium is the printed book – as in the traditional anatomy atlas – or cyberspace, as in the Visible Human Project (Waldby, 2000). Whether book-based or virtual, anatomy does not 'illustrate' bodies so much as it 'demonstrates' them (Waldby, 2000: 91).

In short, much of clinical education, and clinical surveillance and diagnosis, comprises encounters between the clinician and representations of human bodies: for example, the temperature graphs, X-ray images, and electrical traces in the patient record (Berg, 1997; Berg & Bowker, 1997). In these encounters, the patient is no longer necessarily the 'corporeal' person in the bed or on the examining table, but rather the 'hyperreal' re-presentation of that patient on screen in the form of a rhythm strip, black and white picture, colorized image, or digital or other display (Williams, 1997).

Material culture studies is an inter-/trans-/cross-disciplinary and eclectic field of study in which scholars, typically anthropologists, archaeologists, art historians, cultural geographers, cultural studies scholars, folklorists and historians of technology, study physical objects in order to understand history, culture and lived experience. Material culture studies scholars[2] interpret past and present human activity using the physical objects people have left behind or currently use. In addition to quilts, clothes, hospital signs and incubators, the human body itself may be an object of material culture study as human beings have sought to alter and adorn their bodies through body painting and piercing, body building, cosmetic and trans-gender surgery, and reproductive and genetic engineering. Moreover, with the advent of technologies that have made human bodies and body parts more 'plastic', 'bionic', 'interchangeable', and 'virtual', (Williams, 1997), bodies are now themselves indistinguishable from other 'technological artifacts' (Oldenzeil, 1998: 181). Scholars in this highly diverse and expansive field share a general belief that material data can contribute to our understanding of human behavior and values and to what it means to be human, because such materials can be made to reveal the operations of the human mind – its intelligence, imagination, beliefs, and fears. Such materials are assumed to be, and are therefore studied as, historical and 'cultural statements' (Schlereth, 1982: 2; see also Fleming, 1974; Worden, 1993).

Prown (1996: 21) distinguished between hard and soft material culturists.[3] The hard material culturist emphasizes the material side of material culture, or Material culture, while the soft material culturist emphasizes the culture side of material culture, or material Culture. Emphasized in Material culture study is the analysis of the form (e.g. shape, texture, color, special markings), properties (e.g. mechanical, electrical, chemical), internal structure and operations of objects. For example, the study of surgical instruments entails understanding how their design changed with the introduction of surgical asepsis (Edmonson, 1991).

Having some material understanding of objects is necessary for any kind of material culture studies. The very thingness of things shapes, regulates and constrains human behavior and interactions. Pop-ups on computer screens and alarms on monitors force users to address their concerns before users can return to their own work. Infusion pumps regulate the amount of medications a patient can have; in the language of actor-network theory, these pumps serve as delegates for nurses in ensuring patient safety (Prout, 1996: 202). Objects may also 'enforce a morality' (Hodder, 2000: 708) in ways that merely relying on the judgment or beneficence of a human being cannot. Speed bumps curtail speeding in a way that merely posting a speed limit does not, as the practical consequence of speeding over a speed bump is damage to the car.

In contrast, emphasized in material Culture study is the interpretation of how and what objects mean: for example, the metaphors and symbols surrounding objects and how they convey, reinforce, or show resistance to cultural norms, beliefs and/or values. For these material Culturists, artefacts are first and foremost cultural phenomena, shaped not only by scientific, material, and/or economic forces, but, more importantly, by human inclinations and desires. Artefacts become what they are by virtue of what they are physically (which is itself determined by human beings, in addition to such factors as available materials, stylistic conventions and scientific knowledge), and by virtue of what human beings make them out to be.

While Material culturists tend to study objects as technological (arte)facts, material Culturists tend to read them as cultural texts, looking for information about the beliefs, habits, motivations, and desires of their makers and users. Material culturists draw theoretically from materials science and the physical sciences, such as chemistry and physics, and employ quantification techniques and technical analysis to interpret and re-present objects. In contrast, material Culturists employ methodologies oriented to the study of history, culture and personal experience, including semiotics, deconstruction, ethnomethodology and phenomenology. Material culture study is thus methodologically primarily scientific; in contrast, material Culture study is methodologically largely ethnographic and hermeneutic.

Making matter mean

Contributing to the difficulty of making matter mean is that physical objects are highly 'ambiguous' (Lawrence, 1992). So full of meaning are they that they resist simple interpretation. As Kingery (1996) observed, things function as tools, symbols and signs. For example, the computer is 'meaningful' as a physical object comprising hard- and software, as a cultural symbol of or metaphor for an age or *Zeitgeist*, and for the texts and images it contains and produces (Jensen, 1993). The internet, made possible by computers, is both a (cyber)place where culture is formed and a product of culture (Hine, 2000). Accordingly, the 'grammar of things is related to, but more complex and difficult to decipher than, the grammar of words' (Kingery, 1996: 1). Things can be read as technological texts (and computers, as texts within texts), but also as 'myths and poetry' (p. 1). The study of things can get us closer to lived experience, but, like lived experience, they are not easy to articulate (Hodder, 2000).

A key consideration in material culture studies is to discern how objects mean. A pot (or an object we call a pot) does not mean in the same way as the word 'pot'. Most material symbols do not mean in the same way as language – through 'rules of representation' – but rather through 'association and practice' (Hodder, 2000: 707). An object such as a stethoscope has meaning beyond its commonly accepted function in clinical practice: to auscultate heart or other sounds from the interior of the body. Although not designed to be anything but an auscultative device, the stethoscope also communicates and represents status and science. Such objects have been used to promote nursing as a scientific profession to a 'technologically literate audience' prepared to see these objects as symbols of science, which have 'semiotic primacy' in western cultures (Walker, 1994: 52).

The primary concern and problem for any student of material culture is to make 'mute evidence' speak (Hodder, 2000: 703). This objective may appear especially daunting and even contradictory to the qualitative researcher in a practice discipline who typically relies on living persons to speak for themselves. Yet objects also speak, although what they say (like what people say) is not self-evident and may even mislead, without strategies to decipher their meaning and without additional information to place objects in their proper historical and cultural contexts (Lawrence, 1992; Edmondson, 1993). Material culturists have made objects speak by framing them in a variety of methodological frameworks. For example, Tilley (1990) featured structuralism, post-structuralism and hermeneutics as positions from which to 'read' material culture. Feldman (1995) featured ethnomethodology, semiotics, dramaturgy and deconstruction as interpretative approaches for the study of campus housing. Ball and Smith (1992) featured content, symbolist and structuralist techniques, approaches from cognitive and visual anthropology, ethnoscience and ethnomethodology, to study visual data, including photographs, face and body decorations, and print advertisements. Rose (2001) featured compositional, content and discourse analysis, and semiology and psychoanalysis, in her review of visual methodologies. And Schlereth (1982) compared a variety of approaches to the study of American material culture, including art history, symbolism and cultural history; environmentalism, functionalism and structuralism; and behaviorism, national character and social history.

Studies exemplifying these different approaches vary on several parameters, including the kinds of artefact and interpretive objective of primary interest to the researcher, and the research methods employed. For example, environmentalists have typically included cultural and historical geographers and anthropologists with a substantive interest in landscape features, especially housing, and an interpretative interest in space, who use fieldwork methods to study the diffusion of artefacts in a region. Functionalists have typically been historians of technology, folklife scholars, archaeologists, and also cultural anthropologists with a substantive interest in technological systems, and an interpretative interest in the development of technologies, who use fieldwork and experimentation to test the usefulness of objects. Structuralists have typically included folklife scholars, ethnographers with an emphasis on linguistics, and also cultural anthropologists with a substantive interest in vernacular folk housing and popular culture, and an interpretative interest in human consciousness, who use fieldwork to find the grammar of physical data.

Research techniques for studying the material culture of nursing

In summary, a highly diverse range of interpretative positions and methodologies is available to researchers with varying disciplinary commitments and interpretative objectives to study a range of artefacts, including objects of various dimensions, lived environments (e.g. hospitals), living objects (e.g. human bodies) (Emmison & Smith, 2000), and virtual objects (e.g. the internet) (Hine, 2001). And these methodologies may be technically executed in a variety of ways. Studying the material culture of nursing requires an imaginative and eclectic blend of strategies, only a few of which I feature here. The data collection and analysis techniques I describe below seem to be of particular use for nurse researchers, as they can be readily incorporated into and enhance the value of the methodologies they already use, such as phenomenology and ethnography. These techniques entail the cultivation of visual, in addition to verbal, literacy and skills, and an understanding of the highly diverse ways in which credible interpretations are produced and validity is judged.

Ordinary looking

Basic to any approach to the study of things is what Corn (1996: 37) called 'ordinary looking'. Simply paying close attention to objects and other features of the physical landscape of practice will lead to new insights and new questions concerning practice. Why are clocks mounted where they are? Why are the surfaces of some machines slanted as opposed to flat? Why are rooms laid out as they are? Do these positions, surfaces and arrangements influence (e.g. facilitate or constrain) nursing work? Just paying attention to the things around them will lead nurses with an interest in Material culture, engineering skills and knowledge of materials science to deeper physical/technical analyses, with a view toward redesigning the material world of nursing practice to facilitate healing (e.g. Dyson, 1996; Pattison & Robertson, 1996; Kraker & Vajdik, 1997).

Phenomenological reflection

A hallmark of phenomenological reflection is the exquisite study of the concrete, in the service of understanding a universal about the human condition. Indeed, it is the emphasis on the concrete – the corporeal and material – which makes phenomenological reflection so well suited to the study of things as artefacts of lived experience. Kenneth Haltman's (1990) material culture study of a 1923 candlestick telephone demonstrates what can be gained by sensory, intellectual and emotional engagement with objects: by attending to the look, feel and appeal of things, and then by 'empathetic[ally] linking … the … world of the object with the perceiver's world of existence and experience' (Prown, 1982: 8). Philosopher Don Ihde's (1979) work on the human/machine relationship is an excellent example of a phenomenology drawn from first-hand encounters with and contemplation of objects in interaction with bodies. Peggy Anne Field's (1981) 'phenomenological look' at giving an injection addresses a universal contradiction for nurses: namely, that nurses routinely inflict pain in order to relieve it.

Using the 'lifeworld existentials' of corporeality, relationality, spatiality and temporality as guides to phenomenological reflection (Van Manen, 1990: 101), material culturists can gain access to the sensations and visceral emotions involved in actual encounters with objects. For example, I learn about the weight and sharpness of a needle by handling it and pricking myself with it. I learn about the pressure needed to penetrate human tissue with a needle by my (failed) efforts to penetrate human skin. Handling needles not only teaches me about the resistance of the human body to penetration, but also about my own resistance (ability and will) to penetrate it. Knowing these things thus also teaches me something about myself: my manual skills, aesthetic inclinations and anxieties.

Somewhat removed from first-hand familiarity with things, but nevertheless valuable to taking things seriously, is to observe or elicit others' (e.g. patients, family members, colleagues) accounts of their first-hand encounters with things. Such vicarious knowledge is still closer to lived experience than the second-order concepts scholars typically confine themselves to in procedural accounts of physical objects. Phenomenological reflection as a mode of studying material culture is not about – as in the case of needles – gauges, routes of administration, or the physics of tissue resistance (although these are key components of Material culture), but rather about pushing, plunging and holding our breath as we plunge the needle in, feeling a patient's limb move away, or hearing a patient gasp or cry.

In short, knowing patients phenomenologically entails knowing the things nurses use to appraise, treat and comfort them. Another case in point is the ordinary telephone, which nurses are increasingly using as a clinical instrument to appraise and treat patients. Although 'telephone nursing' and 'telephone nurses' now comprise recognized nursing practices and identities (Nauright et al., 1999), nurses have yet to study the telephone itself as a key actor mediating these practices and identities. For example, the telephone enables a kind of 'distance nursing' to occur, whereby nurses and their patients no longer occupy the same space. Tele-nursing calls into question the meaning of 'presence', which nurses have described as central to nursing care (Hines, 1992; see also Swartz & Biggs, 1999). Indeed, the array of tele-encounters now increasingly characterizing health care dramatizes the paradoxes of absent presence and distant closeness (see also Ihde, 1979; Sandelowski, 2001).

Participant observation and fieldwork

An ethnographically informed means to study the material culture of nursing entails varying degrees of participation, from active engagement with objects to observation of others' encounters with them, in a specific field of study. Studying nursing practice mediated by telecommunications technology also entails resolving the challenges raised by efforts to conduct and produce 'virtual ethnographies' (Hine, 2000). Bailey (2000) studied the implementation of a clinical information system in a labor and delivery unit. Key components of her research design included using the new system herself and drawing on her first-hand experiences with paper records, as a basis for comparison. Her study was theoretically framed in the work of information science scholars who view the patient record as a material and cultural tool that structures, facilitates and constrains clinical work, as opposed to the more traditional view of the record as an acultural and immaterial reflection or end-product of work (Berg, 1996, 1997; Orlikowski, 1992). Another key component of Bailey's work was the use of a 'talk aloud' strategy (Fonteyn et al., 1993) to capture what often remains unexpressed as humans engage objects. She used this strategy with herself, and with the clinicians she observed, to verbalize action while in the act. The talk aloud technique can also be used to gain phenomenological access to objects and objects in use, for example to the range of psychomotor activities involved.[4]

Targets of observation

Ethnographic studies of material culture may entail a range of foci or targets of observation. One focus may include verbal interactions with objects. We often talk to the things we use. Most certainly, targets of observation will include non-verbal behaviors. Sometimes, we caress or kick the things we use. And, artefacts have themselves been characterized as a 'mode of nonverbal communication, akin to body language, [or] proxemics' (Prown, 1996: 23). A variety of scholars have used proxemic variables, or measures of the distance and orientations between bodies, to study engagement and readiness to interact amongst people. As things can be viewed as bodies and bodies as things (Williams, 1997), techniques for studying body formations and other nonverbal expressions of communication, interaction and relationship can be usefully applied to the study of material culture (Patterson, 1983; Kendon, 1990; Robinson, 1998; De Roten et al., 1999).

Non-verbal behaviors that comprise important targets of observation include the vocal characteristics of speech, such as loudness, tempo and tone, and a range of proxemic and other variables. Coding systems and rules for interpretation already exist for targeting such factors as the orientation of persons in relation to the objects of study, their respective leans, directions and distance; gestures, hand motions and touch; facial expression; body posture and postural adjustments; foot and leg movements; self and object manipulations; and visual orientation and gaze. One of my students and I found it informative to note how the ultrasound screen was oriented in relation to the sonographer and patient in our study of how nurses use ultrasonography (Huffman & Sandelowski, 1997).

Such observations, collected in person or recorded via videotape and re-presented in visual form (e.g. photos, videos, schematic drawings), can reveal the intimacy, immediacy and tone of interactions, where alliances are drawn, and where impediments to interaction exist. For example, a common truism in nursing is that machines cause nurses to pay less attention to patients. But is this true? And, if true, under what circumstances are machines attended to more than patients? What is the nature and benefit to the patient of this attention? What do machines themselves contribute to encounters between nurses and their patients? What kind of position and power do they have in an interaction *vis-à-vis* the nurse and patient? Is there a place, between nurse and machine and/or machine and patient, to intervene, and is such intervention warranted?

The gaze is a critical non-verbal parameter for observation because so much of clinical work now involves images and screens. The 'visual objectification' of the body, as in X-rays, contributes powerfully to patients' experiences of illness (Rhodes *et al.*, 1999). Drawing primarily from literature in film studies, photography, advertising and cultural studies, where the gaze is a key analytic concept, Chandler (1998a) described forms of gaze (e.g. the bystander, averted, or editorial gaze), the direction of gaze (e.g. toward people, objects, middle distance, the eyes, face, other body part), angles of view, social codes for looking, and other parameters for observation of the gaze. Simon's (1999) ethnographic study of the interaction between images and people in diagnostic conferences illustrates well what can be learned from taking such things as images seriously as material and cultural artefacts. In this study, where participants and images were located in the 'same' place, the images themselves were the central actors. One key finding was the 'vision-oriented hierarchy' (Simon, 1999: 147) revealed in the seating arrangements during the meetings Simon observed. This hierarchy seemed to reflect and reinforce the social hierarchy that already exists in western health care. The diagnostic team's co-directors, a neurosurgeon and radio-oncologist, had unimpaired views of the images projected on screen, while the nurse and technician had to squint to see the details of the images, and non-team members (e.g. house staff) had to crane their necks to see them.

Media/content analysis

Physical objects lend themselves well to analysis as media, where the primary mode of analysis has been quantitative content analysis, and a secondary and emerging mode of analysis is qualitative or ethnographic content analysis (Altheide, 1996). Objects such as X-ray and ultrasound machines and the texts they produce can themselves be usefully conceived of as media and even as mass media (Kevles, 1997; Sandelowski, 1998, 2000).

In contrast to quantitative content analysis of media, in which the researcher systematically applies a pre-existing set of codes to the study of a medium such as newspapers and print advertisements, qualitative or ethnographic content analysis of media is data-derived. Qualitative content analysis is reflexive and interactive as researchers continuously modify their treatment of data to accommodate new data and new insights about that data. Although researchers might also begin the qualitative content analysis process with pre-existing and theoretically driven coding systems, these systems are always modified in the course of analysis, or may even be wholly discarded in favor of a new system, to ensure the best fit to the data.

For example, Stern (2000) explored the homepages that adolescent girls create. A first step was to engage these websites as material artefacts apart from their creators; she plans to conduct online interviews with a selected sample of girls who create homepages. Stern drew from the literature on print media to create a preliminary coding system for analyzing the form and content of these sites, noting such things as color, font size, content of text and pictures, relative space accorded to words as opposed to pictures, and the position of pictures in relation to words. She also included factors distinctive to websites, such as the position and function of links, and the content of the information found in these linked sites. As she collected this data, she modified her coding system to ensure its close fit to the 'thingness' of websites, as they can be read as flat texts and as interactive devices. Stern's initial analysis of the sites themselves, informed by the psychology of color, theories of female adolescent development and modes of self-expression, and western and postmodern constructions of the self, gave her a basis for constructing interview questions that will allow her to understand what girls intended for and by their sites.

Semiotic analysis

In contrast to media/content analysis, semiotics is a more complex, penetrating and controversial mode of cultural analysis and inter-pretation. Semiotics is the study of signs and systems of significa-tion: that is, the study of anything that stands for something else, such as words, images, gestures and objects, and how they come to have meaning in a culture (Chandler, 1998b). Semioticians, amongst whom are linguists, psychoanalysts, cultural anthro-pologists, literature scholars, Marxists and feminists, variously study semantics, or the relationship of signs to what they stand for; syntax, or the relations between signs; and pragmatics, the ways in which signs are used and interpreted. Contemporary semioticians often emphasize the social and ideological uses of signs, finding this form of cultural study valuable for illuminating values, power arrangements, and other taken-for-granted features of everyday life. Semiotic study has features of both symbolic interactionism and ethnomethodology, in that semioticians presume that our relationship with the physical and social world is mediated by symbolic processes, and in that semioticians study the 'rules of use by which communications are produced and interpreted' (Barley, 1983: 7).

Since semiotics is a highly complex mode of study requiring more than a brief section in a chapter to describe fully and well, I feature here some examples of semiotic study that seem especially relevant for nursing inquiry. Barley's (1983: 6) semiotic study of funeral work illustrates how we can usefully conceive of culture as 'shared codes that allow the communication of group-specific interpretations'. Barley studied how funeral work comprises codes for achieving 'naturalness' and 'normality' (p. 11), to offset the sorrow, fear, and even revulsion that westerners often experience around death. Of special note is his detailed analysis of the 'codes of posed features', and 'cosmetic', 'clothing', and 'positioning' codes for making corpses look like living, sleeping persons. A potentially critical application for nursing is in the area of perinatal bereavement, where great pains are taken to give parents material mementoes of life from their dead infants (e.g. locks of hair, nail clippings), in order to offset the cultural tendency to treat perinatal death as a non-event. Moreover, special care is taken to adhere to certain 'rules' for presenting a dead infant – in person and in photographs – in ways that will celebrate its short life, while offsetting the coldness, discolorations and disfigurements of death (Reddin, 1987; Griesbach, 1988; Primeau & Recht, 1994). A key component of the 'sacred and the profane' (Wolf, 1988) in nursing work is the bodily care of the dead, not only of 'dead' corpses, but also of 'living' corpses from whom/which organs will be harvested. Semiotic study can illuminate this highly distinctive and emotionally charged area of nursing practice, and the value of studying bodies as material objects.

In their study of directional hospital signs, Sharrock & Anderson (1979: 81) demonstrated how such material signs can be usefully viewed as 'instances of the socially orderly achievements of practical activities'. Including several photographs of these signs in their report, they proposed that reading signs is an 'embedded activity', that is, 'we read this sign in this way because it is here and because it is next to this other thing' (Sharrock & Anderson, 1979: 90). These signs, variously colored, shaped, sized and positioned, are key but often taken-for-granted features of the hospital landscape that direct movement and help hospital workers, patients and visitors find (and, sometimes, lose) their way.

In her semiotic analysis of campus housing, Feldman (1995) demonstrated the competing meanings of campus housing as 'institutions' and as 'homes'. Her analysis has special significance for the study of the changing geography of health care, which over the twentieth century has moved from home to hospital and back to home again, and now into cyberspace. Infusion pumps, ventilators and other hospital paraphernalia now increasingly populate the home, while 'homey' furniture and room decors now increasingly characterize the hospital. Virtual environments of care are increasingly becoming the rule as clinicians and patients encounter each other over telephone lines and on screen. As in the case of the campus housing Feldman studied, the place of care continues to signal competing meanings related to home and institution, real and virtual space. Material culture studies can contribute to our understanding of the changing physical and moral 'geography' of nursing practice and of sickness (Liaschenko, 1994, 1997).

In my semiotic treatment of the nursing/technology relationship (Sandelowski, 1999), I sought to enhance understanding of this equivocal and even troubled relationship by describing the practices by which nurse/nursing and technology come to stand for and against each other. For example, nurses have been depicted as thermometers and monitors, which, in turn, have been used to stand for nurses/nursing. But such depictions have complicated nurses' efforts to represent nursing also as the caring antidote to the scientific/technical cure embodied in these devices. That is, nurses have variously and sometimes simultaneously sought to align themselves with science and technology, entities highly valued in western cultures, and with feminine caring, an entity devalued in western culture and often depicted as the polar opposite of science and technology. This semiotic treatment of the nursing/technology relationship offers another reason why nurses continue to have difficulty constructing nursing as different from medicine and mere 'womanly' practices.

Material culture studies and nursing

In conclusion, material culture studies can lead nurses to the 'right' questions to ask and to answers to some of the 'big questions' (Lubar, 1996: 31) that address nursing as a distinctive set of material and embodied practices. Nurses also have a special contribution to make to the study of material culture by virtue of the embodied practices that distinguish nursing from all other practice disciplines. Learning directly from things, and from things in use, will return nurses to valuing and using the body as 'a tool' (Short, 1997: 9), not merely for practice, but also for research; it is the fully embodied self that is the key instrument in conducting qualitative studies of distinction and significance for nursing (Savage, 2000).

Notes

1. Different cultures draw different lines between people and objects. Moreover, in the turn-of-the-twentieth-first-century world of bionic people, vital machines and artificial intelligence, the line between person and object is harder to draw (Pickstone, 1994; Sandelowski, 2000).
2. The kinds of scholar I mention may not necessarily think of themselves as material culturists. I use the term here in the most generic sense to include any discipline that concerns itself with people in interaction with things.
3. The designations 'hard' and 'soft' unfortunately reinforce a gender-coded hierarchy, according to which hard study is considered more objective and truer than soft study. As I vehemently object to such designations, I avoid these terms in my subsequent discussion of material culture studies while remaining faithful to Prown's meaning.
4. In the actual practice of research, methods are more dynamically interrelated and artfully used than they appear in research textbooks, where rigid lines are typically drawn between methodological approaches such as phenomenology and ethnography. After all, research 'design' implies an artistic endeavor as much as a scientific one. Any individual study might have elements of more than one methodological approach. A largely ethnographic study might have phenomenological overtones, while a largely phenomenological study might have cultural overtones. I believe that any 'good' qualitative study is characterized in part by some attention to culture, history and lived experience.

References

Altheide, D.L. (1996) *Qualitative Media Analysis*. Thousand Oaks, CA: Sage.Atkinson, P. & Silverman, D. (1997) Kundera's *Immortality*: the interview society and the invention of the self. *Qualitative Inquiry* 3: 304–25.

Ball, M.S. & Smith, G.W.H. (1992) *Analyzing Visual Data*. Newbury Park, CA: Sage.

Bailey, D. (2000) *Nurse work and the computerized patient record*. PhD dissertation, University of North Carolina at Chapel Hill.

Barley, S.R. (1983) The codes of the dead: the semiotics of funeral work. *Urban Life* **12**: 3–31.

Berg, M. (1996) Practices of reading and writing: the constitutive role of the patient record in medical work. *Sociology of Health and Illness 18* **4**: 499–524.

Berg, M. (1997) Of forms, containers, and the electronic medical record: some tools for a sociology of the formal. *Science, Technology and Human Values* **22**: 403–33.

Berg, M. & Bowker, G. (1997) The multiple bodies of the medical record: toward a sociology of an artifact. *Sociological Quarterly* **38**: 513–37.

Bijker, W.E., Hughes, T.P. & Pinch, T.J. (eds) (1987) *The Social Construction of Technological Systems: New Directions in the Sociology and History of Technology*. Cambridge, MA: MIT Press.

Callon, M. (1995) Four models for the dynamics of science. In S. Jasanoff, G.E. Markle, J.C. Petersen & T. Pinch (eds) *Handbook of Science and Technology Studies*. Thousand Oaks, CA: Sage, pp. 29–63.

Chandler, D. (1998a) Notes on 'the gaze'. Available on line at [www.aber.ac.uk/~dge/gaze.html] Retrieved 12/27/99.

Chandler, D. (1998b) Semiotics for beginners. Available on line at [www.aber.ac.uk/media/Documents/54B/Semiotic.html] Retrieved 10/27/99.

Channell, D.F. (1991) *The Vital Machine: A Study of Technology and Organic Life*. New York: Oxford University Press.

Chasin, A. (1995) Class and its close relations: Identities among women, servants, and machines. In J. Halberstam & I. Livingston (eds) *Posthuman Bodies*. Bloomington, IN: Indiana University Press, pp. 73–96.

Corn, J.J. (1996) Object lessons/object myths? What historians of technology learn from things. In W.D. Kingery (ed) *Learning From Things: Method and Theory of Material Culture Studies*. Washington, DC: Smithsonian Institution Press, pp. 35–54.

Csikszentmihalyi, M. & Rochberg-Halton, E. (1981) *The Meaning of Things: Domestic Symbols and the Self*. Cambridge: Cambridge University Press.

De Roten, Y., Darwish, J., Stern, D.J., Fivaz-Depeursinge, E. & Corboz-Warnery, A. (1999) Nonverbal communication and alliance in therapy: the body formation coding system. *Journal of Clinical Psychology* **55**: 425–38.

Dunlop, M.J. (1986) Is a science of caring possible? *Journal of Advanced Nursing* **11**: 661–70.

Dyson, M. (1996) Modern critical care unit design: nursing implications in modern critical care unit design – bed area ergonomics. *Nursing in Critical Care* **1**: 194–7.

Edmonson, J.M. (1991) Asepsis and the transformation of surgical instruments. *Transactions and Studies of the College of Physicians of Philadelphia* **13**: 75–91.

Edmonson, J.M. (1993) Learning from the artifact: surgical instruments as resources in the history of medicine and medical technology. *Caduceus* **9**: 87–95.

Emmison, M. & Smith, P. (2000) *Researching the Visual*. London: Sage.

Feldman, M.S. (1995) *Strategies for Interpreting Qualitative Data*. Thousand Oaks, CA: Sage.

Ferguson, E.S. (1977) The mind's eye: nonverbal thought in technology. *Science* **197**: 827–36.

Field, P-A. (1981) A phenomenological look at giving an injection. *Journal of Advanced Nursing* **6**: 291–6.

Fleming, E.M. (1974) Artifact study: a proposed model. *Winterthur Portfolio* **9**: 153–73.

Fonteyn, M.E., Kuipers, B. & Grobe, S.J. (1993) A description of think aloud method and protocol analysis. *Qualitative Health Research* **3**: 430–41.

Griesbach, S.J. (1988) A medical photographer's role on a perinatal bereavement team. *Journal of Biological Photography* **56**: 149–53.

Haltman, K. (1990) Reaching out to touch someone? Reflections on a 1923 candlestick telephone. *Technology in Society* **12**: 333–54.

Hamilton, D. (1994) Constructing the mind of nursing. *Nursing History Review* **2**: 3–28.

Haraway, D.J. (1991) *Simians, Cyborgs, and Women: The Reinvention of Nature*. New York: Routledge.

Hayles, N.K. (1993) The materiality of informatics. *Configurations: A Journal of Literature, Science, and Technology* **1**: 147–70.

Hine, C. (2000) *Virtual Ethnography*. London: Sage.

Hines, D.R. (1992) Presence: discovering the artistry in relating. *Journal of Holistic Nursing* **10**: 294–305.

Hodder, I. (2000) The interpretation of documents and material culture. In N.K. Denzin & Y.S. Lincoln (eds) *Handbook of Qualitative Research*, 2nd edn. Thousand Oaks, CA: Sage, pp. 703–15.

Huffman, C.S. & Sandelowski, M. (1997) The nurse–technology relationship: the case of ultrasonography. *Journal of Obstetric, Gynecologic and Neonatal Nursing* **26**: 673–82.

Ihde, D. (1979) *Technics and Praxis: A Philosophy of Technology*. Dordrecht, Holland: D. Reidel.

Jensen, J.F. (1993) Computer culture: the meaning of technology and the technology of meaning. A triadic essay on the semiotics of technology. In P.B. Andersen, B. Holmqvist & J.F. Jensen (eds) *The Computer as Medium*. New York: Cambridge University Press, pp. 292–336.

Kendon, A. (1990) *Conducting Interaction: Patterns of Behavior in Focused Encounters*. Cambridge: Cambridge University Press.

Kevles, B.H. (1997) *Naked to the Bone: Medical Imaging in the Twentieth Century*. New Brunswick, NJ: Rutgers University Press.

Kingery, W.D. (1996) Introduction. In W.D. Kingery (ed.) *Learning From Things: Method and Theory of Material Culture Studies*. Washington, DC: Smithsonian Institution Press, pp. 1–17.

Kouwenhoven, J.A. (1982) American studies: words or things? In T.J. Schlereth (ed.) *Material Culture Studies in America*. Nashville, TN: American Association for State and Local History.

Kraker, K. & Vajdik, C. (1997) Designing the environment to make bathing pleasant in nursing homes. *Journal of Gerontological Nursing* **23**: 50–51.

Latour, B. & Woolgar, S. (1986) *Laboratory Life: The Construction of Scientific Facts*. Princeton, NJ: Princeton University Press.

Lawler, J. (1991) *Behind the Screens: Nursing, Somology, and the Problem of the Body*. Melbourne: Churchill Livingstone.

Lawrence, G. (1992) The ambiguous artifact: surgical instruments and the surgical past. In C. Lawrence (ed.) *Medical Theory, Surgical Practice: Studies in the History of Surgery*. London: Routledge, pp. 295–314.

Liaschenko, J. (1994) The moral geography of home care. *Advances in Nursing Science* **17**: 16–26.

Liaschenko, J. (1997) Ethics and the geography of the nurse–patient relationship: spatial vulnerabilities and gendered space. *Scholarly Inquiry for Nursing Practice* **11**: 45–59.

Lubar, S. (1996) Learning from technological things. In W.D. Kingery (ed.) *Learning from Things: Method and Theory of Material Culture Studies*. Washington, DC: Smithsonian Institution Press, pp. 31–4.

Lynch, M. (1985) Discipline and the material form of images: an analysis of scientific visibility. *Social Studies of Science* **15**: 37–66.

Moore, L.J. & Clarke, A.E. (1995) Clitoral conventions and transgressions: graphic representations in anatomy texts, c. 1900–1991. *Feminist Studies* **21**: 255–301.

Nauright, L.P., Moneyham, L. & Williamson, J. (1999) Telephone triage and consultation: an emerging role for nurses. *Nursing Outlook* **47**: 219–26.

Oldenziel, R. (1996) Objections: technology, culture, and gender. In W.D. Kingery (ed.) *Learning From Things: Method and Theory of Material Culture Studies*. Washington, DC: Smithsonian Institution Press, pp. 55–69.

Oldenziel, R. (1998) Review of Bernice L. Hausman's *Changing Sex: Transsexualism, Technology, and the Idea of Gender*. *Technology and Culture* **39**: 179–81.

Orlikowski, W.J. (1992) The duality of technology: rethinking the concept of technology in organizations. *Organization Science* **3**: 398–427.

Orr, J.E. (1996) *Talking About Machines: An Ethnography of a Modern Job*. Ithaca, NY: ILR Press/Cornell University Press.

Parker, J. (1997) The body as text and the body as living flesh: metaphors of the body and nursing in postmodernity. In J. Lawler (ed.) *The Body in Nursing*. Melbourne: Churchill Livingstone, pp. 11–29.

Patterson, M.L. *Nonverbal Behavior: A Functional Perspective*. New York: Springer-Verlag.

Pattison, H.M. & Robertson, C.E. (1996) The effect of ward design on the well-being of post-operative patients. *Journal of Advanced Nursing* **23**: 820–26.

Pickstone, J. (1994) Objects and objectives: notes on the material cultures of medicine. In G. Lawrence (ed.) *Technologies of Modern Medicine*. London: Science Museum, pp. 13–24.

Primeau, M.R. & Recht, C.K. (1994) Professional bereavement photographs: one aspect of a perinatal bereavement program. *Journal of Obstetric, Gynecologic, and Neonatal Nursing* **23**: 22–5.

Prout, A. (1996) Actor-network theory, technology and medical sociology: an illustrative analysis of the metered dose inhaler. *Sociology of Health and Illness* **18**: 198–219.

Prown, J.D. (1982) Mind in matter: an introduction to material culture theory and method. *Winterthur Portfolio* **17**: 1–19.

Prown, J.D. (1996) Material/Culture: can the farmer and the cowman still be friends? In W.D. Kingery (ed.) *Learning from Things: Method and Theory of Material Culture Studies*. Washington, DC: Smithsonian Institution Press, pp. 19–27.

Reddin, S.K. (1987) The photography of stillborn children and neonatal deaths. *Journal of Audiovisual Media in Medicine* **10**: 49–51.

Rhodes, L.A., McPhillips-Tangum, C.A., Markham, C. & Klenk, R. (1999) The power of the visible: the meaning of diagnostic tests in chronic back pain. *Social Science and Medicine* **48**: 1189–203.

Robinson, J.D. (1998) Getting down to business: talk, gaze, and body orientation during openings of doctor–patient consultations. *Human Communication Research* **25**: 97–123.

Rose, G. (2001) *Visual Methodologies*. London: Sage.

Rudge, T. (1999) Situating wound management: technoscience, dressings and 'other' skins. *Nursing Inquiry* **6**: 167–77.

Sandelowski, M. (1998) Looking to care or caring to look? Technology and the rise of spectacular nursing. *Holistic Nursing Practice* **12**: 1–11. Erratum in **13** (1): 82–4.

Sandelowski, M. (1999) Troubling distinctions: a semiotics of the nursing/technology relationship. *Nursing Inquiry* **6**: 198–207.

Sandelowski, M. (2000) *Devices and Desires: Gender, Technology, and American Nursing*. Chapel Hill: University of North Carolina Press.

Sandelowski, M. (2001) Visible humans, vanishing bodies, and virtual nursing: Complications of life, presence, place, and identity. Manuscript submitted for publication.

Savage, J. (2000) Participative observation: standing in the shoes of others? *Qualitative Health Research* **10**: 324–39.

Schlereth, T.J. (1982) Material culture studies in America, 1876–1976. In T.J. Schlereth (ed.) *Material Culture Studies in America*. Nashville, TN: American Association for State and Local History, pp. 1–75.

Sharrock, W.W. & Anderson, D.C. (1979) Directional hospital signs as sociological data. *Information Design Journal* **1**: 81–94.

Short, P. (1997) Picturing the body in nursing. In J. Lawler (ed.) *The Body in Nursing*. Melbourne: Churchill Livingstone, pp. 7–9.

Silverman, D. (1998) Qualitative research: meanings or practices? *Information Systems Journal* **8**: 3–20.

Simon, C.M. (1999) Images and image: technology and the social politics of revealing disorder in a North American hospital. *Medical Anthropology Quarterly* **13**: 141–62.

Stafford, B.M. (1994) *Artful Science: Enlightenment Entertainment and the Eclipse of Visual Education*. Cambridge, MA: MIT Press.

Stern, S. (2000) Making themselves known: Girls' WWW homepages as virtual vehicles for self-disclosure. PhD dissertation, University of North Carolina at Chapel Hill.

Swartz, J.D. & Biggs, B. (1999) Technology, time, and space or what does it mean to be present? A study of the culture of a distance education class. *Journal of Educational Computing Research* **20**: 71–85.

Tilley, C. (ed.) (1990) *Reading Material Culture: Structuralism, Hermeneutics and Post-Structuralism*. Oxford: Basil Blackwell.

Trachtenberg, A. (1979) *Brooklyn Bridge: Fact and Symbol*, 2nd edn. Chicago: University of Chicago Press.

Van Manen, M. (1990) *Researching Lived Experience: Human Science for an Action Sensitive Pedagogy.* Albany, NY: State University of New York Press.

Waldby, C. (2000) *The Visible Human Project: Informatic Bodies and Posthuman Medicine.* London: Routledge.

Walker, K. (1994) Confronting 'reality': nursing, science and the micro-politics of representation. *Nursing Inquiry* **1**: 46–56.

Wiener, C., Strauss, A., Fagerhaugh, S. & Suczek, B. (1997) Trajectories, biographies, and the evolving medical technology scene: labor and delivery and the intensive care nursery. In A. Strauss & J. Corbin (eds). *Grounded Theory in Practice.* Thousand Oaks, CA: Sage, pp. 229–50.

Williams, S.J. (1997) Modern medicine and the 'uncertain body': from corporeality to hyperreality? *Social Science and Medicine* **45**: 1041–49.

Wolf, Z.R. (1988) *Nurses' Work: The Sacred and the Profane.* Philadelphia: University of Pennsylvania Press.

Worden, G. (1993) Steel knives and iron lungs: medical instruments as medical history. *Caduceus* **9**: 111–18.

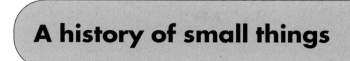

CHAPTER 11

A history of small things

Siobhan Nelson

'History is always parable to the truth. The truth is always there but in some other form than we might expect. The truth is there with the same qualities with which we experience it in everyday life – sometimes uncertainly, sometimes contradictorily, sometimes clouded by the forces that drive us to it, sometimes so clearly that it blinds us to anything else.' (Dening, 1996: 1)

Questions of truth and meaning haunt every methodological discussion. Here too, I will bravely address these questions as we examine historical approaches to the subject of nursing, and explore the nursing profession's particular relationship with historical discourse. The chapter commences with an examination of the methodological debates within history on truth and constructivism, and the moves to discuss the possibilities offered by emergent trends in historiography that illuminate social practice, technologies and power. Nursing work is often cloaked in simplicity. It is argued here that historians of nursing need to consider the small tasks involved in everyday nursing procedures, they need to notice the mundane and humble artefacts of such work – the pan, the sluice, the saline, the draw sheet or the cotton ball. In this way, what nurses did, as opposed to what nursing represented can be revealed. Finally, by way of illustration, I take these philosophical and methodological quandaries to the analysis of historical data from a single Melbourne archive to examine nineteenth-century nursing practice. Throughout the chapter the aim is to promote a complex and sophisticated idea of historical sensibility as a prerequisite to undertaking historical research, and to counter trends within nursing scholarship that generate conventional readings of nursing history.

'What is history?' is the perennial epistemological and methodological question for historians. Definitions abound and are always contested. The answer can never be straightforward. Rather, this question engenders a discussion on the purpose of history and its place in contemporary scholarship. For the most part, historians would agree that good history makes its reader see things differently. It brings into view a world or set of events in a surprising way, challenging the certainties of the present, complexifying the taken-for-granted conceptions of the past. But it is clear, too, that history can serve any purpose – from propaganda to nostalgia to subversion. Let us, then, direct the question 'what is history?' to the specifics of nursing history, to examine its purpose and its capacity to make us see things differently.

Nursing history

Paradoxically, nursing is both the subject of and the producer of historical narrative. Nurses and historians engage in writing nursing history. Surprisingly, these two enterprises need scarcely intersect. As the subject of historical scholarship, nursing provides a rich field for women's history, for the history of practice and the professions, for labour history, and for the history of technology and science. For their part, nurses have long produced nursing history as a vital element in the professional armoury. The narrative of nursing leaders-turned-historians constructed nursing in a particular way – as a story of steady progress towards the light. Thus one finds a home-grown nursing history rehearsing tales of nursing's centrality to the evolution of the health care system and of its vital importance to a humane society – nursing's own 'grand narrative'.[1]

But, as the Australian historian Greg Dening observed, 'A history that is seen to believe its own fictions is a fraud and bore. It loses moral force on both scores' (Dening, 1996: 3). Freed of nursing fictions, all kinds of intellectual pursuit become possible within the boundaries of history. Consider the raw material. The hospital of the nineteenth and twentieth centuries was powered by nurses. Nursing labour cared for patients, delivered babies and laid out bodies, managed technology, coordinated departments, ran admissions, discharges and home care; controlled the operating room – theatres, list and procedures; recycled, cleaned, repaired and packed dressings, gloves, linens; maintained instruments and machines; wrote and maintained patient records; managed the kitchen, the domestic staff and the laundry (the engine rooms of the hospital). The hospital hummed with nursing labour 24 hours a day, 365 days a year. These (mainly) women worked and lived in the hospital for years, even spending their entire working lives in a single institution. Much of the work that nurses did was carried out away from the patient eye, taking place in the sluice room, the drug room, the procedure room or operating theatre. The private and invisible world of nursing, a world known only to initiates, mysterious to patients and overlooked by medicine, contained practices and knowledges never mentioned in public.

Beyond the hospital walls, the trained nurse occupied a paradoxical place in society – lowly and elevated. As a private duty nurse, the nurse's work collapsed the boundaries between wife, mother, nurse and servant, and she paid the price for this ambiguity. In the homes of others, the nurse was totally responsible for the patient's care (without relief) and exploited as a domestic worker (McPherson, 1996). On the other hand, as a public health figure the nurse represented both feminine authority and the power of the state (Buhler-Wilkerson, 1987). The social impact of the trained nurse was remarkable. The nurse pioneered careers for women in the military and even evangelised as missionaries throughout the world. She was a vital figure in many a rural community and the leading female player in health service bureaucracies. The possibilities for nursing history, then, burst from the page – flowing through the stories of nurses' lives and work is the history of gender, of race, of technology, of power and the professions. Yet is this the nursing history we know?

The power and the glory of the nursing narrative

Much of what we think we know about nursing today, and how we imagine the past, has been mediated by the received narrative of nursing history. Traditionally nursing leaders took up their pen and set down the truth. It was a powerful history that had 'filtered out intractable problems' (James, 1984). It wrote into being the importance of nursing by trained women as a female remedy to a vast array of physical and social ills (Nelson, 1997, 2002). It was a tonic for nurses and ammunition for the great battles they fought, and fight to this day, for respect and power. These narratives formed part of the history of the profession that nurses embraced in their training school curricula. The function of this work, then and now, was to foster a sense of nursing's tradition, to emphasise the break with the old and the gains of new. It was the onwards and upwards kind of history that pleased its subjects – the commissioning institution or association (Nelson, 2002).

The place of history in nursing discourse changed dramatically when nursing transferred from the training schools to the universities. In the university a new set of imperatives operated on the nursing curricula. Instead of importance being attached to the traditional history of nursing in one's hospital, state or country, the locus of authority was transferred from the alumni, and the profession generally, to the academy (Nelson, 1997). With knowledge development in the tertiary sector and the generation of the nursing as a discrete discipline, nurses interested in history began to conform to the imperatives of the new dominant discourse in nursing – not the professional progressivist narrative of the old leaders, but the progressivist narrative of knowledge development. Somewhat belatedly, British nursing historian Christopher Maggs responded to this displacement of the role of history in nursing by calling for historians to make their work relevant to this disciplinary project through a history of caring (Maggs, 1996). Meanwhile in the USA, as a fresh young discipline, nursing had begun to cement its rules. One of the fundamentals agreed upon by nursing scholars was the creation of 'nursing-specific knowledge' (Fawcett, 2000). Nursing scholarship, as a stand-alone discipline, adopted qualitative methodologies as a minor element of the nursing science project. And it was under this umbrella that history became reborn in nursing as a 'legitimate research method for nursing' (Sarnecky, 1990).

History as a method

Nursing theorist Teresa E. Christy pioneered history as a qualitative method in nursing in the 1970s (Christy, 1975, 1981). It is curious how history was snatched up in this way, regularised and formatted into a set of discrete steps and adapted to fit an uncontested set of universal laws of validity. Examples of the enduring currency of this recipe approach are not hard to find – let two stand for many. According to the standard research method text by Polit and Hungler (now in its sixth edition):

> 'Historical research is the systematic collection and critical evaluation of data relating to past occurrence. Generally, historical research is undertaken to answer questions concerning causes, effects, or trends relating to past events that may shed light on present behaviours or practices.' (Polit & Hungler, 1999: 248)

Compare this view with John Tosh's: 'History is an inventory of possibilities, all the richer if research is not conducted with half an eye to our immediate situation' (Tosh, 2000: 20). In addition to the 'presentist' focus of nursing history as a qualitative methodology, a concept we will return to shortly, this approach is characterised by an unproductive preoccupation with the concept of validity. In a second popular research methods text (now in its fourth edition), LoBiondo-Wood and Haber claim that 'establishing fact, probability and possibility with the historical method' is quite straightforward. A fact is established when

> 'two independent primary sources agree with each other, or one independent primary source that receives critical evaluation and one independent secondary source that is in agreement and receives critical evaluation and no substantive conflicting data.' (LoBiondo-Wood & Haber, 1998: 234)

There are two critical issues in this convoluted attempt to legitimate historical scholarship as research method under the nursing lexicon: first, the preoccupation with 'fact' and 'bias' is anachronistic, rendered irrelevant by the post-structuralist debates of recent decades. But more importantly, there is no mention in these method guides to the connection between historical data and the social context – the very task of history. This was the problem identified by James in her 1984 review essay on nursing history in which she observed of one case of historical research produced from within nursing:

'Overall, however, no structure of interpretation, no explanation of historical changes, no significant comparisons or
conclusions emerge from this densely factual account, not even
on the theme of professionalization announced in the subtitle
or introduction. Perhaps the difficulty is the author's meagre
knowledge of the history of medicine and public health (the
nineteenth century sanitary movement for example) and the
history of women; the context for her research is missing.'
(James, 1984: 576)

History is neither a collection of facts nor a set of rules for data
validity. It is the interplay between historical data and the fusion of
narrative and analytical writing. History as a 'method', therefore,
emerges as something of an orphan – sitting uncomfortably within
nursing scholarship – with its contrived facts and validity, and
resting apart from mainstream historical scholarship that would
complicate and enrich it.

But as already discussed, nurses are not the only producers of
historical narrative on nursing and we are greatly indebted to the
social historians who have interested themselves in the professions,
engendering a cross-fertilization of insights, preoccupations and
approaches (Burnham, 1998). Two decades ago, social historians
and nursing historians together began to look at nursing in a more
complex way. As a result of this trend, the 1980s was an aston-
ishing decade of revision and critique of the traditional nursing
narrative. For once, everyone was interested in nursing – it was a
topic of substance exciting the imagination of the likes of Davies
(1980), Melosh (1982), Tomes (1984), Vicinus (1985), Reverby
(1987), Dingwall *et al.* (1988), Poovey (1988), Summers (1988,
1989), amongst others. These researchers, immune to the holy
imperatives of nursing history, situated their nursing history within
women's history, social history and labour history. They took
advantage of the enormous source material and extraordinary
stories nursing can provide, and at the same time explained the
social and gender context of nursing's story to nurses (Nelson,
2002).

In addition to the work of these 'outsider' historians, nursing has
also been blessed by the work of nursing scholars who are trained
historians (Nelson, 1999a). These writers bring an outsider's

method to the insider's view, and as a result they possess that rare gift – a historical sensibility combined with an intimate eye. Historians such as Maggs (1983), Baly (1986, 1987), Lynaugh (1988, 1989), Helmstadter (1993, 2001), Rafferty (1996), D'Antonio (1999) are amongst the nursing historians who have contributed enormously to the insider–outsider richness of nursing history. Not only have these scholars spoken to nurses of their practice and history, they have also (and this is critical) communicated the story of nursing to historians of medicine, historians of women, labour historians and social historians – all the areas of scholarship with which nursing history does and must intersect. This scholarship, however, is unable to fulfil the criteria espoused by Jacqueline Fawcett, that research must produce 'nursing-discipline specific knowledge' (Fawcett, 2000: 525), for these nursing historians eschew a nursing framework, relying instead on historical rigour and sophisticated narrative. Their work is not qualitative research but wonderful history.

Methods and means

But nursing is not alone in its battles over disciplinary truths and the nature of knowledge. It could be argued that historians have been more troubled by postmodern critiques than even their besieged colleagues in the sciences. Facts are seldom uncontested in history and, in the end, interpretation is all – a parade of signifiers with the reader writing the text, as Roland Barthes contentiously claimed (Barthes, 1981), or as Bryant termed it, 'a fabulatory product of the present'[2] (Bryant, 2000: 490). And even if some facts withstand the onslaught of deconstruction (an atomic bomb destroyed Hiroshima on 9 August 1945), they stand like lonely islands in a sea of confusion (did it cause the Japanese to surrender?).

On examination, most of the historical facts that constitute the collective narratives of our social world do not stand close scrutiny. Let us take for example one of the best-known stories in nursing history, Florence Nightingale and the reform of nursing. The person in the street or the average nurse will tell you Nightingale invented modern trained nursing (I have polled this response myself on countless occasions). Few historians would claim this. In fact,

Monica Baly showed that Nightingale was very unhappy with both St Thomas' Hospital Training School and the matron Mrs Wardroper. The great Nightingale Model was created by a series of political contingencies, and took a form that rarely pleased her (Baly, 1986, 1987). Moreover, my own research examines the enormous influence of nursing nuns, Catholic and Anglican, on Nightingale's views on nursing and argues that her 'invention' was very much a repackaging and promotion of an idea already in circulation (Nelson, 2001a).

What about the regulation of nursing? This event is always heralded as the great breakthrough for progress. Was it? In Britain, many have argued that regulation handed power from nursing, which was self-regulating to some degree, to the state, and British nursing has been very much dominated by government ever since (Rafferty, 1996: 184). In Australia, perfectly good systems of self-regulation were passed over to a series of politically controversial boards in the (vain) pursuit of political influence on the part of the nursing leadership (Nelson, 1999b). In the USA, Reverby tells us, registration was directly linked to the extension of power and influence of the elite schools of nursing (Reverby, 1987). History can be reassuring; good history can be disturbing. If Florence Nightingale did not create modern nursing, what did she do and why is she so important? If registration legislation was not the dawn of the new age of light and progress, why was it so hard fought? These unsettling questions are vital precisely because they are unnerving.

Nursing history, however, has traditionally been constructed in a reassuring mode. To see beyond its comfort zone reveals a different world. For instance, as D'Antonio (1999) argues, if one begins with the social history of women who worked as nurses, and resists the urge to privilege their professional lives over their lives as mothers, women or community members, a very different history of nursing (and women) emerges. Similarly, the complex religious history of nineteenth-century nursing has been rendered invisible by the narrative of the secular nurse reformers. This rewriting has been so successful that, today, religious nurses of the past are not even recognised as nurses. But once one sees beyond this narrow narrative, the lives of many hundreds of thousands of religious women in the old and new worlds come into focus, and with that so many elements of contemporary nursing – such as its vocational ethos and its gendered form – begin to make sense (Nelson, 2001b).

So what is truth and what are facts? This is the question that all researchers must answer, or at least take a position on. For the historian, the answer to this question provides philosophical orientation for the research, it gives the researcher a track on which to move from the archive to the secondary literature, to the narrative under construction. Let us take two examples of methodological orientation. First, a progressive account of science, medicine and nursing. This account assumes that things are better now than back then, that knowledge has developed, and with that development professional training and patient care have much improved. Underpinning this view – unstated and unvisited – is a belief in what Lyotard (1984) so dismissively described as the Enlightenment Project. That is the view that knowledge and progress improve and enlighten the human condition. This is the view staunchly defended by Fukuyama (1992). Fukuyama and others have fought back against the relentless onslaught of relativism, deriding its intellectual fashions and posturing – daring, even at the end of the twentieth century – to draw lines between fact and fiction (Burns, 1994).

For our second example let us take the Foucauldian approach. This perspective could be interested in a number of topics – power, the body, surveillance and so forth. For instance, it may examine the relationships between the technology the nurse uses, surgical techniques and the development of a 'professional space'. These relationships emerge as helping to constitute the nurse as a professional – they exemplify the knowledge–power nexus to professional evolution. Underpinning this perspective is a particular stance on both truth and history. Foucault argued that truths were constituted within an episteme, he sought to explore the taken-for-granted or self-evident and was interested in continuities and discontinuities in historical narrative (Foucault, 1990). For Foucault history did not necessarily move forward, though the perception that it did so was an important taken-for-granted element of asymmetrical distributions of knowledge/power relations.

Both of these views are somewhat extreme and do not divide historical scholarship to the extent that one may think. In fact, good historians have never been confused by the issue of truth. They have long understood the role of selectivity, active interpretation and tracing of narrative that occurs, and how the story becomes powered by its own logic. As E.H. Carr wrote in 1961, long before any postmodern assault on truth was born,

> 'the belief in a hard core of historical facts existing objectively and independently of the interpretations of the historian is a preposterous fallacy, but one which is very hard to eradicate.' (Carr, 1961: 30)

In recent years historians have expressed their frustration at the empirical historian 'straw man' that is under endless attack by postmodernists (Karnstein, 1993: 520). As Stone remarked: 'hyperconstructionism scores most of its points against an imaginary opponent' (Stone, 1992). Moreover, defenders of old 'grand theory', such as historians Eley & Nield, rebut postmodern attacks on Marxism theory arguing that 'Surely we can see real events occurring behind people's backs without reaffirming the entire conceptual lexicon of problematic structuralism?' (Eley & Nield, 1995: 359).

While historians have been sceptical about Foucault's methodological competence (he was, it must be admitted, a poor historian), many have nonetheless been stimulated by his notions of discourse, his views on power, his genealogical method and the idea of 'historicisation', that is the manner in which objects or ideas become themselves the subject of history (Foucault, 1990). This work has provided historians with tools and a vocabulary for thinking about historical narrative and the present in stimulating and provocative ways.

A history of the present

Contemporary questions require a particular type of history, a history which looks back to 'shed light on how contemporary practices function' (Castel, 1994: 244), to challenge the self-evidence and 'demonstrate the precariousness' of historical processes (Foucault, 1991: 75). This type of history is underpinned by a view of the present as 'a moment that is traversed by the flow of multiple temporalities and the descent of multiple processes which are traced by several histories' (Dean, 1994: 33). To trace these histories requires a genealogical analysis, a process which 'interrogates the past from the vantage point of the needs and complexities of the present situation' (Goldstein, 1994: 14). A genealogy is not a history of an evolutionary process through which the rational becomes real. Genealogy produces a mapping of the threads that constitute the present. While it may provide a narrative of events, it is not a subject-centred account (Nelson, 2000). Thus the picture that emerges is one of 'serial histories' (Dean, 1994). In my own work, *A Genealogy of Care of the Sick* (Nelson, 2000), I set out to explore the connection between care of the sick and ethical practice. I was interested in how the care of strangers became constituted as 'good work' and the implications of this history on contemporary nursing as an ethical practice. Using the ideas of askesis and governmentality (explored by Foucault in his late work on self-culture), I mapped the history of care of the sick as a virtue from early Christian times to the present.

Further influential strands in historiography include cultural history, an approach heavily indebted to Geertz's anthropological 'thick description' (see, for instance, Geertz, 1983; Darnton, 1984; Hunt, 1989). Sandelowski's work demonstrates the value of this approach to the creation of a cultural history of nursing (Sandelowski, 2000). Anthropological perspectives can provide insights into the technological basis of practice, examines the knowledge and skill basis of practising nurses, and analyse the emergence of 'expertise' in discrete areas of clinical practice.

Postcolonialism is another increasingly influential theoretical trend in history. Postcolonialism represents a set of theories that unleash race and gender critiques of world history and reconstruct narrative from the perspective of the colonised. It has turned on its head the adage that victors write history (Shohat, 1992; Moore-Gilbert, 1997). This approach has enormous untapped potential for nursing history. I am currently engaged in researching a history of Australian nursing that views the Nightingale movement and its enduring legacies as a form of colonialism, and explores the ethnic and racial implications of this English nursing model for the development of nursing and health services in Australia.

But how much has history changed in the light of these arresting intellectual developments, and what do they mean for nursing history? It appears that what remains standing after decades of debate is a history 'unnerved [if unconvinced] by postmodern posturing against the empirical' (Bryant, 2000: 494). It is a more cautious discipline, one concerned with subtlety and complexity, nervous of ambit claims, causes and truths. There are at least two implications for nursing history. First, the gap between the discipline of history and much nursing scholarship is set to widen if nursing continues to use history as a device to support the old grand narrative of progress and legitimacy – what Lucien Febvre called 'the deification of the present with the aid of the past' (Febvre, *Combats pour l'histoire*, 1933, cited in Jones, 2000: 533). A second, happier possibility is that nursing researchers will re-examine the 'truths' of nursing history and rewrite the narrative full of richness and possibility – without the inevitability, without the great women, without nursing as a part of the great leap forward.

To the archive . . . ways to rewrite a history of nursing

Nurse Archer

Let us take as a case study some 110-year-old clinical notes from the Royal Women's Hospital Archive, the case of Mrs S and Nurse Archer:[3]

'In 1890, twelve months after she had become pregnant, Mrs S was admitted to the Women's Hospital, Melbourne, with an abdominal pregnancy. Surgery removed the foetus, leaving intact the cyst, and parts of the placenta and sac that were adhered to the bowel wall. This was to undergo decomposition postoperatively.

Week 1   Following surgery Mrs S's great pain and restlessness was settled with one quarter of a grain of morphia given every few hours. Dark bloody fluid was drawn off the cyst via a glass drain, which was then irrigated with Mercuric chloride 1–300 tds. Mrs S was treated with nourishing enemata of milk and egg, brandy and champagne were given freely by mouth. Mrs S's temperature rose and fell dramatically, peaking each night. Her pulse and respirations were rapid. Flatus was treated with enemas... Day 5, diarrhoea was controlled with chalk and opium.

Week 2   The cyst, by now black, had begun to slough off. Towards the end of the week an abscess had formed on the suture line. The wound was washed in Condy's solution. Mrs S's diarrhoea remained and she was treated with Quinine. Stimulants, nourishment and hot water bottles were given frequently.

Week 3   Mrs S developed a severe pain in the calf of her left leg. The leg was raised and poulticed and morphia recommenced. Mrs S's condition deteriorated. She was 'very low', passing urine involuntarily. Roused only with stimulants and great care.

Week 7   Nurse Archer, who had been nursing this case day and night since the operation, having refused relief, developed a slight attack of pleuro pneumonia... "She completely broke down and had to be removed and kept in bed for some time. She left the case in good condition."

Week 17   Four months following the operation Mrs S discharged home.'

This summary of a richly detailed account of the intimate care of a critically ill woman plunges us into the history of nursing practice. Much of this account is familiar to any trained nurse. From a distance of 110 years one can imagine giving Mrs S pain relief, attending to the painstaking dressings, sedating her. Her moans, her dry mouth and sharp breath; the bed baths, and the tiny sips of fluid and soothing pieces of ice are all utterly familiar elements of the sick room. But much of the story confuses or even astounds us. No contemporary nurse could understand fever as Nurse Archer did (fever management is one of the lost arts of nursing). How was a deep vein thrombosis managed prior to anticoagulant therapy? The complicated administration of brandy and champagne, and nourishing enema are equally perplexing. What form did the champagne come in? Were they popping corks at the bedside?

Whatever the science behind this medicine or the logic of the nursing, it is clear that this woman owed her life in the first place to her surgeon's skill, but in no lesser part to the postoperative care provided by Nurse Archer. But how is it possible to make sense of the tale of Nurse Archer's heroic care? A traditional and tempting approach would be to claim it. It could be argued that nursing retains those selfless elements, that her efforts were part of nursing's true heritage that formalised with nursing reform when nurses became trained and regulated. It is not possible to know precisely Nurse Archer's training but it is conceivable she was a respectable woman with two years' training (McCalman, 1998: 78). It could be argued that modern nursing worked to make Nurse Archer the rule not the exception, and Nurse Archer was in fact the personification of the new reformed nurse. This narrative reinforces the profession's noble history and reasserts many of the values that nursing holds dear to itself. However, this approach would also invite reproach as whiggish, anachronistic or presentist. Whiggish history

> 'underestimates the differences between past and present – [it] projects modern ways of thought backwards in time and discounts those aspects of past experience alien to modern ideas'. (Tosh, 2000: 120)

Presentism is the greatest pitfall of history written by enthusiasts. Scrupulous attention to the accuracy of the historical record will not protect the writer from this fate if they lack a sophisticated sense of historical context. What, then, are some other possibilities?

Nurse Archer's behaviour could be explored from the question of nursing as an emerging profession. Nurse Archer's refusal to hand over care, her dramatic collapse once her patient was out of danger are scarcely the models for a regularised and consistent system of scientific nursing. To bring reform, stability and predictability to the bedside it may have been necessary to discipline heroics such as those of Nurse Archer.[4] In this sense, then, Nurse Archer is interesting because she is located at what Foucault would call a moment of rupture (Foucault, 1997). This is a significant time when one discursive form or set of structures is overtaken or reconstituted for another. Nurse Archer may be written as a continuity – claimed for the noble nurse of the future – or she may be constructed as an outmoded form – the outstanding amateur – soon to be vilified by the reformers in their campaign for trained nurses.

Other accounts of nursing care from the nineteenth-century archive that produced Nurse Archer are equally enthralling. In McCalman's compelling history of the Women's Hospital in Melbourne (McCalman, 1998), we find that surgical vaginal repairs in the late nineteenth century, for appalling degrees of bladder or bowel prolapse and perineal tears, were performed upon conscious women, tied into an all-fours position for the procedure and for their postoperative nursing care. These innovative surgical techniques were breakthroughs, but it was the preoperative and postoperative nursing care that made the difference between the transformation of the woman's life or continued misery. In some of these cases the woman required ten weeks preoperative preparation. The woman would be admitted to be nourished and rested. Her ulcerated and infected perineum was kept clean with irrigations and dressings so that the tissue could repair to a sufficient state to allow surgery. Postoperatively, the woman was kept sedated and constipated by opium tincture, and catheterised intermittently via glass urethral catheters (by medical staff). Success depended upon the wound site remaining clean of urine and faeces. Once the sutures were removed and the wound healed, the woman was weaned off the opium and assisted to gradually manage her bodily functions unaided. This was intensive and skilled nursing by any measure. But how is it possible to reconstruct this skilled nursing? What training did the nurses receive? What implements did they use? What did they chart? The commonsense idea that nurses have increased their clinical skill may be disabused by a study of the practice of nurses past. No doubt, contemporary nurses are more technologically competent but this cannot be conflated with clinical skill. From the archive it is possible to reassemble surgical nursing in the final three decades of the nineteenth century. Surgical success and the emergence of skilled surgical nurses are but one story that rises from these records. Other possibilities include the rise and fall of the now defunct speciality of gynaecological nursing.

The final suggestion lends itself to a Foucauldian style historicisation of the place of 'profession' in nursing. It is possible to examine these records with a mind to the notion of profession, when it was first introduced, how it was used and what it meant. This is more than an analysis of language. The professional discourse has had enormous power in nursing and would be particularly suitable for historicisation in this way. Not only are ideas and concepts suitable subjects for historicisation, but practices and objects can also be fruitful subjects of analysis. Oral histories, stock lists, procedure manuals and student curricula provide the data for just such a reconstruction of practice. Oral histories are invaluable but perilous, and the historian must be aware of the rehearsed nature of the subject's life story (Silverman, 1998). In my own experience of elderly ex-military nurses, the women wished only to relate their favourite stories of indiscipline, camaraderie or student nurse horror story. Mundane questions prove enormously difficult for subjects to answer. They, too, find it hard to recall the daily routine of the ward – a topic so unimportant for so long. Yet historicising objects and practices demands this attention to the mundane and the creative use of sources such as stock lists, photographs or examination papers. Concentrating on the history of small things reveals breaks in our everyday understanding of nursing history and identity.

Conclusion

Nursing has long produced a noble narrative, both through the nursing leaders of the past and more latterly as the historical arm of nursing science. This history unproblematically constructs a narrative that moves from darkness to light. It shows the inevitability of progress through the timely interventions of strong and insightful leaders. But freed of these linear imperatives what shapes appear? What form does the story of nursing begin to assume without the 'great women' of nursing history? What are the lives that nurses led? What did they actually do? What effect has nursing, with its troubled professional, political and resolutely *gendered* history, had on the lives of women? On the health care system? On medicine? What has been the story of nursing for North American women? British women? African women? For there is no *one* story of nursing, but countless stories of women (and some men) and their lives of work and practice.

Work and practice: these must be the starting point for rich and revealing histories of nursing. Imagine, for example, tracing cotton wool balls to reconstruct a story about nursing. But such historical adventures must be free from the tyranny of the nursing narrative. They must not seek to prove or validate the importance of nursing or be burdened with responsibility for the reconstruction of history as a nursing-specific discipline. There is no fundamental truth about nursing that must be revealed – heroic tales or stories of repression alike. Rather, let us explore small things – the practices, artefacts and tasks of nursing. Let us also explore the partial and contingent manner in which a mass profession for women emerged, its vagaries and delusions, its power and achievement.

Notes

1. For illustrations of the grand professionalising narrative see for instance, Nutting & Dock, 1907; Seymer, 1932; Stewart & Austin, 1962; Goodnow, 1963.
2. Bryant was depicting 'the other side' here, his own views reassert historical validity.
3. This cameo is constructed from notes and records held by the Royal Women's Hospital Archive. The story of Mrs S and Nurse Archer features in Janet McCalman's, *Sex and Suffering*, 1998, 73–8.
4. I am grateful to Janet McCalman for discussions on this point. McCalman also raised some of these issues in her paper 'The power of care: "special" nursing 1880–1910', *Women's Bodies/Women's History*, University of Melbourne, 21–23 June 2001.

References

Baly, M.E. (1986) *Florence Nightingale and the Nursing Legacy*. London: Croom Helm.

Baly, M. (1987) The Nightingale nurses: the myth and the reality. In C. Maggs (ed.) *Nursing History: The State of the Art*. London: Croom Helm, pp. 33–59.

Barthes, R. (1981) The discourse of history. *Comparative Criticism* 3: 7–20.

Bryant, J.M. (2000) On sources and narratives in historical social science: a realist critique of positivist and postmodern epistemologies. *British Journal of Sociology* 51 (3): 489–523.

Buhler-Wilkerson, K. (1987) Left carrying the bag: experiments in visiting nursing, 1877–1909. *Nursing Research* 36: 42–7.

Burnham, J.C. (1998) *How the Idea of Profession Changed the Writing of Medical History*. London: Wellcome Institute for the History of Medicine.

Burns, T. (ed.) (1994) *After History? Francis Fukuyama and his Critics*. Lanham, MD: Rowman & Littlefield.

Carr, E.H. (1961) *What is History? The George Macaulay Trevelyan Lectures delivered in the University of Cambridge, January–March 1961*. London: Macmillan.

Castel, R. (1994) Problematisation and reading history. In J. Goldstein (ed.) *Foucault and the Writing of History*. Oxford: Blackwell.

Christy, T.E. (1975) The methodology of historical research: a brief introduction. *IMAGE: Journal of Nursing Research* **4** (3): 189–92.

Christy, T.E. (1981) The need for historical research in nursing. *IMAGE: Journal of Nursing Research* **11**: 227–8.

D'Antonio, P. (1999) Revisiting and rethinking the rewriting of nursing history. *Bulletin of the History of Medicine* **73**: 268–90.

Darnton, R. (1984) *The Great Cat Massacre and Other Episodes of French Cultural History*. New York: Basic Books.

Davies, C. (ed.) (1980) *Rewriting Nursing History*. London: Croom Helm.

Dean, M. (1994) *Critical and Effective Histories: Foucault's Methods and Historical Sociology*. London: Routledge.

Dening, G. (1996) History's theatre. *Australian Humanities Review*, July, pp. 1–4.

Dingwall, R., Rafferty, A.M. & Webster, C. (1988) *An Introduction to the Social History of Nursing*. London: Routledge.

Eley, G. & Nield, K. (1995) Starting over: the present, the post-modern and the moment of social history. *Social History* **20**: 359.

Fawcett, J. (2000) Editorial: But is it *nursing* research? *Western Journal of Nursing Research* **22** (5): 524–5.

Foucault, M. (1990) *History of Sexuality, Vol. 2, The Use of Pleasure*. London: Penguin.

Foucault, M. (1991) A question of method. In G. Burchell, C. Gordon & P. Miller (eds) *The Foucault Effect: Studies in Governmentality*. Chicago: University of Chicago Press.

Foucault, M. (1997) *The Archeology of Knowledge*. London: Routledge.

Fukuyama, F. (1992) *The End of History and the Last Man*. New York: Free Press.

Geertz, C. (1983) *Local Knowledge: Further Essays in Interpretative Anthropology*. New York: Basic Books.

Goldstein, J. (ed.) (1994) *Foucault and the Writing of History*. Oxford: Blackwell.

Goodnow, M. (1963) *History of Nursing* (rev. by J.A. Dolan). Philadelphia: Saunders.

Helmstadter, C. (1993) Robert Bentley Todd, St John's House and the origins of the modern trained nurse. *Bulletin of the History of Medicine* **67**: 297–302.

Hunt, L. (1989) (ed.) *The New Cultural History*. Berkeley: University of California Press.

James, J.W. (1984) Writing and rewriting nursing history: a review essay. *Bulletin of the History of Medicine* 58: 568–84.

Jones, A. (2000) Word *and* deed: why a *post* poststructuralist history is needed and how it might look. *The Historical Journal* 43 (2): 517–41.

Karnstein, W. (1993) Hayden White's critique of the writing of history. *History and Theory* 32 (3): 273–95.

LoBiondo-Wood, G. and Haber, J. (1998) *Nursing Research Methods, Critical Appraisal, and Utilization*. St Louis, MO: Mosby.

Lynaugh, J.E. (1988) Narrow passageways: nurses and physicians in conflict and concert since 1875. In N.M.P. King, L.R. Churchill & A.W. Cross (eds) *The Physician as Captain of the Ship: A Critical Reappraisal*. Dordrecht: D. Reidel, pp. 25–37.

Lynaugh, J.E. (1989) *The Community Hospitals of Kansas City, Missouri, 1879–1915*. New York: Garland.

Lyotard, J.P. (1984) *The Postmodern Condition: A Report in Knowledge*. Manchester: Manchester University Press.

Maggs, C. (1983) *The Origins of General Nursing*. London: Croom Helm.

Maggs, C. (1996) A history of nursing: a history of caring. *Journal of Advanced Nursing* 23: 630–35.

McCalman, J. (1998) *Sex and Suffering: Women's Health and a Women's Hospital – The Royal Women's Hospital, Melbourne, 1856–1996*. Carlton, Vic.: Melbourne University Press.

McPherson, K. (1996) *Bedside Matters: The Transformation of Canadian Nursing, 1900–1990*. Toronto: Oxford University Press.

Melosh, B. (1982) *'The Physician's Hand': Work, Culture and Conflict in American Nursing*. Philadelphia: Temple University Press.

Moore-Gilbert, B. (1997) *Postcolonial Theory: Contexts, Practices, Policies*. London: Verso.

Nelson, S. (1997) Reading nursing history. *Nursing Inquiry* 4: 229–36.

Nelson, S. (1999a) Insiders and outsiders in writing history, in *A question of ethics: Personal perspectives*. Carlton: History Institute, Vic. Inc., pp. 38–45.

Nelson, S. (1999b) Déjà vu and the regulation of nursing. *Australian Journal of Advanced Nursing* 16 (4): 29–35.

Nelson, S. (2000) *A Genealogy of Care of the Sick*. Southsea, Hants: Nursing Praxis International.

Nelson, S. (2001a) *'Say Little, Do Much': Nurses, Nuns and Hospitals in the Nineteenth Century*. Philadelphia: University of Pennsylvania Press.

Nelson, S. (2001b) From salvation to civics: care of the sick in nursing discourse. *Social Science and Medicine* 53 (9): 1217–25.

Nelson, S. (2002) A fork in the road: nursing history versus history of nursing. *Nursing History Review* 9.

Nutting, M.A. & Dock, L. (eds) (1907) *A History of Nursing. From the Earliest Times to the Present Day with Special Reference to the Work of the Past Thirty Years.* 4 vols. New York: G.P. Putnam's & Sons.

Polit, D. & Hungler, B. (1999) *Nursing Research: Principles and Methods.* Philadelphia: Lippincott.

Poovey, M. (1988) *Uneven Developments. The Ideological work of Gender in Mid-Victorian England.* Chicago: University of Chicago Press.

Rafferty, A.M. (1996) *The Politics of Nursing Knowledge.* London: Routledge.

Reverby, S.M. (1987) *Ordered to Care. The Dilemma of American Nursing, 1850–1945.* Cambridge, MA: Cambridge University Press.

Sandelowski, M. (2000) *Devices and Desires: Gender, Technology and American Nursing.* Chapel Hill: University of North Carolina Press.

Sarnecky, M.T. (1990) Historiography: a legitimate research methodology for nursing. *Advances in Nursing Science* 12 (4): 1–10.

Seymer, L.R. (1932) *A General History of Nursing.* London: Faber & Faber.

Shohat, E. (1992) Notes on the post-colonial. *Social Text* 31/32: 99–113.

Silverman, D. (1998) Qualitative research: meanings or practices? *Information Systems Journal* 8: 3–20.

Stone, L. (1992) Dry heat, cool reason: historians under seige in England and France. *Times Literary Supplement*, 31 January.

Summers, A. (1988) *Angels and Citizens: British Women as Military Nurses, 1854–1914.* London: Routledge & Kegan Paul.

Summers, A. (1989) The mysterious demise of Sarah Gamp: the domiciliary nurse and her detractors, c. 1830–1860. *Victorian Studies* 32 (3): 365–86.

Stewart, I.M. & Austin, A.L. (1962) *A History of Nursing from Ancient to Modern Times: A World View*, 5th edn. New York: Putnam.

Tomes, N. (1984) 'Little world of our own': the Pennsylvania Hospital Training School for Nurses, 1895–1907. In J. Leavitt (ed.) *Women and health in America: Historical Readings.* Madison: University of Wisconsin Press, pp. 467–81.

Tosh, J. (2000) *The Pursuit of History: Aims, Methods and New Directions in the Study of Modern History.* Harlow: Longman.

Vicinus, M. (1985) *Independent Women. Work and Community for Single Women, 1850–1920.* Chicago: Chicago University Press.

CHAPTER 12

Studying the women in white

Joanna Latimer

In this final chapter I focus on several aspects of my ethnography of an acute medical unit in a prestigious UK teaching hospital (Latimer, 2000a). The study took place at a time just before the radical reforms of the UK National Health Service in the 1990s and in a sense anticipates some of the effects of these reforms. One aim of the book is an 'evocation' (Tyler, 1986) of nursing life in contemporary health care services, and practising nurses' responses to talks about the study suggest that it does indeed resonate with their experiences.

The approach in *The Conduct of Care* (Latimer, 2000a) brings issues of identity together with those of power/knowledge. As I researched nurses' conduct I read widely in sociology, anthropology and social theory. Soon I found I began to ask different kinds of questions to those posed by mainstream nursing research. Rather than seeing nurses as failing to live up to set ideals, I asked what was nurses' conduct accomplishing? And why were nurses accomplishing these matters rather than others? That is, what are the wider socio-cultural effects in which nurses are embedded? And how does their conduct help reaccomplish those effects? In asking these kinds of questions my topic, the assessment and care of older people in an acute medical unit, began to emerge as a site of critical interest, to nursing and to sociology.

As discussed in earlier chapters, a field is not a given but is constructed as a site. May (this volume) urges a reflexive awareness of how our approach to the field has distinct political effects. Importantly, we have also stressed that a site is much more than sets of functional practices. Rather, a site is 'made up' of the 'conditions of possibility' (Foucault, 1976) under which nurses practise and which their practices help reproduce. Nelson in her chapter (this volume) showed how a critical historical approach can help illuminate how the present is a site underpinned by ideas and attitudes sedimented over time. In contrast, my approach was to do an ethnography of present practice but in what I understood to be a critical location.

In what follows, I show how we can examine and understand nursing practice in all its complexity. I suggest how to situate nurses' conduct, not just in relations with patients but in all their relations, both strategic and everyday. In order to do this I suggest we have to get 'inside nursing'. This means *finding* nursing in the complex interplay between cultural materials and social practices. The approach offered is not the only approach that can be taken to study nursing, or any other domain of social life for that matter, but it is especially useful for illuminating what nurses accomplish and why.

Constructing a field: occasions for nursing

Taking the assessment and care of older people as my focus, I had put my finger on something of political interest, to governments, to professionals and to older people themselves. This is because in the acute medical domain the status of older people *and* of nurses is precarious, so that my topic was certainly a focus for examining the complex politics of contemporary health care. But it was the ways in which I approached my chosen topic that helped illuminate nurses' assessment and care of older people as 'a site'.

My objective was not to describe nurses' behaviour and then attempt to evaluate how older people were assessed and cared for against some preconceived notion about their medical or nursing needs. This is because I do not think this approach is underpinned by an adequate representation of how nursing occurs: nurses do not simply identify needs and give care, or not. This would be to reduce them to rational-cognitive rather than social beings. Rather, as my study proceeded my objectives extended.

At the same time as I created 'thick descriptions' (Geertz, 1983) of nurses' conduct, I also began to want to understand 'occasions for nursing' as *social* phenomena which have to be explained (cf. Garfinkel and Sacks, 1986). To put it another way, as I went about my ethnographic work of creating thick descriptions of how nurses conducted occasions for nursing, I began to want to be able to *explain* why nurses conducted 'occasions' for nursing in the ways in which they did. For example, I wanted to understand why one staff nurse told me during a morning shift that she did not conduct her care of an elderly woman in line with procedures directed at preserving dignity because she did not have time, while later on in the same shift I saw her making time for the medication round.

Let me recapitulate here. I could have gone along with how many nursing theorists imagine nurses' behaviour. By seeing nurses' behaviour as a matter of knowledge, individual choice, or of group dynamics, theorists limit explanation of good practice or of 'deviations' from good practice, rather than consider how practice connects to nurses' socialness. Where the social in nursing research is incorporated it is often marginalised through, for example, suggesting that nurses' behaviour is merely mimetic or attributable to the effects of the structural properties of institutions.

In contrast, I want to hold on to the idea of conduct, rather than behaviour. The term 'conduct' suggests that the ways in which nurses act and speak reflect aspects of the social. Specifically, the term 'conduct' helps keep in mind that what nurses do helps to organise the world, but not in any way that they please. Rather they are, like all social beings, *conduits* through whose doing and being particular power effects are produced and reproduced.

We can 'see' this aspect of conduct in the ways in which nurses, such as the staff nurse already mentioned above, privilege some kinds of patients or work over others. But we can only understand what it is that they are privileging if we attend to what these moments are made to mean. For example, what is it about the medication round, and what is it about the old woman that gave staff nurse the permission to privilege the medication round over the old woman's dignity? So we need to construct a research approach that enables us to follow through such moments. But we need to be able to follow them not just to their meanings and their effects, although these are important things to understand. Crucially, we need to be able to understand how *staff nurse* knows[1] what and who to privilege and when. We need to be able to identify where *she* gets her permissions from. So the question arises how can we go about 'knowing' what she knows?

The social, then, has to be understood as about *being* social.

Social life is being imagined as the product of interaction rather than individual choice or cognition. But in order to *explain* nurses' conduct the research needs to encompass all possible points of influence in nurses' work and lives. In order to 'find' these key points of influence, the researcher needs to 'get inside' nursing life.

Identity: the priority of membership

The approach I am pressing presumes that to understand nursing practice there is a recognised need to 'go inside'. In making this stand, my own work joins other ethnographies of organisation to take the mundane and the taken for granted seriously because it is through the mundane and taken for granted, as well as the strategic, that meanings are circulated. So in doing participant research the researcher must get inside – but inside whose or what part? How does an ethnographer locate herself? We have already heard about critical issues of self and others in the context of participant observation from Savage and Gerrish (both this volume), but I want to press further the issue of *what* do we want to get inside.

Our concern in this chapter is less with issues of theory and more with making explicit the methods of researching the kinds of reality imagined here. Specifically, one of the ways in which we can 'observe' how social actors together make up reality is through examining their social practices. A crucial social practice in a Euro-American context is the giving of accounts (Garfinkel, 1967). Giddens (1984), drawing on Schutz, states that, in their accounts, actors not only draw upon stocks of knowledge to '*go on*', in their everyday interactions, they draw upon these same stocks of knowledge to make sense of their actions (and the actions of others), to 'make their accounts, offer reasons' (p. 29). 'Stocks of knowledge' involve the 'interpretative schemes' which are the 'modes of typification' which actors use to constitute meaning (p. 29) and are implicated in the communication of meaning. Giddens suggests that while the communication of meaning in inter-actions is to a certain extent governed by the 'structural ordering of sign-systems' (p. 30), 'signs exist only *as the medium and outcome of communicative processes in interaction*' (p. 31, emphasis added).

Thus displaying knowledgeability over interpretative schemes and modes of typification is how social actors 'do member' (Garfinkel, 1967), but the meanings that things have has to be produced and reproduced through their use. Members thus perform identity through their participation in those communicative processes which produce and reproduce sign systems. This means that we can begin researching social life by examining how people organise their world through modes of typification, including categories, such as 'social' or 'medical', 'acute' and 'chronic'. But we need to go a bit further: we need to be able to identify what it is that they make these typifications mean. As Garfinkel (1967), in his breaching experiments demonstrates, it may take a moment of deviance to provoke a situation in which taken-for-granted or implicit meanings can come into view. But in many ordinary situations, such as for the staff nurse discussed above, matters are not so settled. There are always multiple possibilities, so that knowing how and when to align with one way of doing or seeing rather than another, is more complex.

While we can begin to know what it is that people like staff nurse know through paying attention to their social practices, such as the giving of accounts (Munro, 1996a), we need to know *how* she knows what to privilege and when. So that what we need to be able to unpack is *how* it is that she knows what to privilege and when, for example a medication round over an old woman's dignity.

Getting inside: following cultural materials

I want to suggest that we can find a way to get inside by following nurses' key cultural materials. It is not enough simply to follow nurses around. Rather than shadowing the main actors, as other ethnographers have done before us we need to find another way to get inside nursing life. Sandelowski and Nelson (both this volume) have justified paying attention to the materials that nurses make and use. But what are nurses key cultural materials? And how can we follow them?

On arrival in a Balinese village, Geertz (1993) finds that he is invisible: despite being the guest of the village chief, the local people look through him as if he is so much air. This state of affairs goes on for a few weeks, and Geertz thinks he never will be able to get inside the life of the Balinese village that he and his wife have come to study. One night he is intrigued by the idea of attending a cockfight. This is partly because cockfights are banned, and partly because everywhere he goes he has seen Balinese men sitting around talking about, and fondling, their cockerels.

In the middle of the fight there is a police raid. Geertz and his wife, despite being illustrious guests, join the villagers and flee, heaving themselves over a wall into someone's yard. By the time the police arrive, Geertz and his wife are sitting sipping tea with members of the household. When asked, they deny any knowledge of the cockfight. The next day everyone that Geertz passes in the street acknowledges him, smiling and making jokes: the strange anthropologist shifts from being invisible to being included.

From then on, Geertz continues to follow not the Balinese as such, but their cockerels. He follows cockerels through all the practices which the Balinese participate in around them. These practices define cockerels' significance and include all aspects of how the Balinese care for their cockerels as well as the organisation of the fights themselves.

In his analysis, the love and care of cockerels and of cockfighting emerge as a marginal space – it is in-between the old orders of Balinese life and the new Republican demands for civilised society, which includes banning cock fighting, to high days and holidays. But the love and care of cockerels and the organisation of cock fights constitutes a space in which many different layers of Balinese society intersect and interact. At the same time as it is highly ordered and organised, the domain which the care of cockerels and which cockfighting makes up, reflects and helps to reproduce the organisation of Balinese society. Geertz makes vivid that this space is possible only because it is engendered by and engenders extreme and ambiguous emotions. Put baldly, the practices which make up the space of cockfighting are critical because it is through them that Balinese people perform their distinctiveness and thereby the (re)ordering of the Balinese domain. Specifically cockerels and cockfighting help the Balinese to keep in play all the ambivalence which make them distinctive. What emerges is that very little about the Balinese is ever completely settled.

Geertz did not go to Bali expecting to make cockerels and cockfighting so central: his entry was haphazard, it was not planned in any way. Anthropologists before him had studied much less mundane activities, such as religious rites. But it his focus on cockerels, and on all the practices that go on around cockerels and cockfighting, that helps Geertz to get inside the ambiguities and tensions which make up Balinese, as opposed to any other kind of, life.

Cockerels are key cultural materials for the performance of Balinese identities in all their heterogeneity and complexity.[2] Nurses work on, talk about, observe and interact not with cockerels but with patients and with other people also concerned with patients. Patients rather than cockerels are nurses' cultural material. Patients are nurses' key extensions. This is not to suggest that one discourse makes up the identity of a patient: the meanings patients have for nurses have to be produced through discourses and other practices of distinction. There are flesh-and-blood patients' whom nurses handle, touch, serve, administer, speak with, ignore and move around. And there is also the virtual patient made up of nurses' and others' representations of them, composed of systems of distinction. And rather than the living, breathing patient simply defining the virtual patient, the virtual patient's identity to some extent constitutes how nurses conduct their interactions with the living, breathing patient.

The in-between

In order then to get inside nursing life and understand all the points of influence on nurses' conduct, we need to follow patients, not nurses. Focusing on the work of caring for and distinguishing patients gets inside nursing, because it is through this work that nurses perform their identity and keep their world in order. But one needs to find a place from which to follow patients through all of nurses' practices and through all the points of influence upon these practices. In a hospital, this place is the bedside.

In travelling to the patient's bedside I was able to locate myself at the margins and intersections of many aspects of life in hospital. Doctors, nurses, and many others all come to the bedside, encountering the patient as well as each other. In focusing on the bedside's of older people, I put my finger on, like Geertz, a margin between old orders and new, and between contradictory agendas for conduct. The new included increased demands for enhanced visibility and efficiency which older people in their complexity can risk. But also within this view, the bedside as a space from which to administer and care for patients is increasingly constituted as banal and mundane. Relatives, domestics and care assistants are meant to operate at the bedside of care, not professional nurses. Professional nurses are supposed to perform themselves as decision makers at the nurses' station – poring over notes and charts, or staring into screens. At the same time, however, professional calls to nurses imply the potentially contradictory demand for an extended kind of health care – more patient-centred, holistic and individualised. So how do nurses' settle these apparently contradictory agendas? One way is for them to go to the bedside, not with washbowls or bandages, but with a new kind of technology, the nursing process, materialised in forms to be filled in and charts to be displayed.

In my ethnographic work, then, I travel, like an anthropologist, but not to the inside of a mud hut or to a tent in the Sahara, but to the bedsides of patients. At the bedside I sit and wait: observing what flows to and from the patient, noting when and how it flows. This flow includes people (such as nurses and doctors), and other materials[3] (such as food, charts, forms to be filled in, chairs, drugs and machines). What flows from the bedside are excreta, and parts of patients (such as blood samples or pots of spittle), as well as the 'virtual patient' constituted by nurses, doctors and others' representations of them. I follow the virtual patient through all their translations (Callon & Latour, 1981; Callon, 1986) at doctors' ward rounds, nursing handovers, case conferences, and in nursing and medical records. Critically I trace what and who authorises the flow of materials to and from the bedside. It is in these accounts that one can find *what* has authority, *what* gives permission to privilege one kind of work or one kind of patient over another.

The bedside thus lies in between many facets of hospital life. Nurses too lie in between these different facets. The move to the bedside thus helps to make explicit what is usually implicit: that nurses do not have only one part to play. Rather they are themselves situated in between many parts, many agendas and many occasions. And they have to work hard to know how to settle matters.

Figuring patients, performing identity

Patients are nurses' key materials for the performance of identity and through these performances nurses help to reorder their world. But patients, as cultural materials, have to be 'made to mean' (Sandelowski, this volume). Their symbolic value cannot be taken for granted and their meaning does not simply travel from one context to the next. Sandelowski suggests ways in which the researcher can understand what materials are made to mean. For example, following Douglas and Isherwood (1980) we can understand what materials mean through examining how they are talked about and used.

I want to press the idea that in a world where meanings are unsettled, materials have to be made to mean, their meanings are not implicit and cannot be taken for granted. The meanings that materials are made to have must be continuously accomplished and, sometimes, where meanings are contested, settled.

The virtual *and* the fleshy patient are key performative materials for nurses. But nurses, in order for patients to be expressive of their identity, have to *make* patients have symbolic meanings. A patient's distinctiveness is not given.

We can identify how patients are made to mean things through examining the practices of distinction which nurses draw on to 'figure' patients (cf. Latimer, 1997b). For example,

Sister   I do tend to leave the geriatric long-term patients to really middle grade nurses with an auxiliary ... second years, or occasionally first years, depending on the quality of students we have.

Researcher Why, how do you make that sort of decision? What do you base that on?

Sister   Well, I tend to think that even most of the junior nurses know what basic nursing care is. They tend to know how to wash people, feed people, dress and just sit and listen to the older ladies. And they, I would suspect, would probably be a bit more frightened to look after somebody who's got central lines, IVs [intravenous infusions] although they do get an opportunity to do that as well, with the staff nurse.

In this account, the sister is justifying her distribution of the resources at her disposal. Here, then, we are seeing how the flow of resources is authorised. Within contemporary health care this, the justification for the distribution of resources, is central to member's work. For the sister, the resources at her disposal include grades of nurse as well as the things that they do and use. She justifies the ways in which she distributes these resources through associating different kinds of work with different grades of nurse. By a process of association, washing and dressing people is made to seem less difficult than activities concerned with medical technology, such as IVs and central venous lines. In this way, materials such as those connected to washing and dressing (clothes, soap, flannels, washing bowls, baths and showers), are all distinguished as of less importance than technical or clinical materials (such as IVs and central venous pressure lines). Similarly, by association, the identity of one category of patient – 'long-term geriatrics' – is being figured. Those patients such as long-term geriatric who only need bathing and washing, rather than medical technology, are downgraded.

The symbolic meaning of different patients and different categories of patient is accomplished through these kinds of processes of association. By association, materials such as patients' virtual identities are made to mean at the same time as they give meaning. Nurses perform their identity not just through talk but also through the materials they work with because of the meanings they make these materials have. To be simplistic for a moment, one of the ways in which nurses perform a hierarchy is through the kinds of material they are permitted to use and work with, as we can see from the quote from Sister above. The kinds of patient a nurse is permitted to work with helps signify the nurse's identity in the hierarchy. But the meanings which patients are made to have are themselves continuously accomplished through nurses' practices of distinction, such as Sister's above.

In performing these hierarchies nurses, like Sister, are of course drawing upon what is already prefigured (Strathern, 1992): the asymmetrical relation between technology and other kinds of cultural material. Drawing on this relation is what makes Sister's move effective. But in doing this, Sister is reproducing it, and helping to (re)order the world. In this instant then, at the same time as she helps to give nurses identity, she aligns[4] with, and remakes (see also

Latour, 1986), a world in which personal care signifies the banal and mundane, while the technological is elevated to the heroic. Where these kinds of 'move' are in circulation across many differently situated occasions, we begin to know what Staff Nurse at the beginning of the chapter knows. And we can begin to understand why she privileged the medication round over the dignity of the old woman. The old woman was a 'long-term geriatric'.

Unsettling times

I have stressed the need for research methods that get us inside nursing. What I have problematised throughout this chapter is that how we imagine social life affects the question of what it is that we want to get inside. In this penultimate section I want to draw out more of the interconnections between social theories and the practice of research.

My title makes reference to a seminal study of medical students. *The Boys in White* (Becker *et al.*, 1961) was a 1950s study coming out of the interactionist Chicago school of social science. In making this reference I want to connect my own approach to the interactionist perspective on how social life is produced: but only up to a certain point. For Becker (1993), becoming a doctor was shown to be as much about a process of socialisation as it was about getting to grips with medical knowledge and skills. Within this view of socialisation, the medical students want to be seen to belong, and in order to do so they learn and follow the social rules and conventions which underpin the medical domain. Behaviour is thus explained as more about learning and following the rules and routines of social life than it is about being rational. The difficulty here is that social actors emerge as what Garfinkel (1967) calls cultural dopes: being social in this view of socialisation is too rigidly conceived as about learning the conventions as somehow fixed and 'out there', and 'knowing' all about when to follow and when to deviate.

While the idea of conduct is also based on a theoretical tradition that has as its starting point that persons are not free do whatever they will, it incorporates a notion that social organisation depends for its coherence on people *participating as persons*. Indeed, as

Garfinkel (1967) suggests, it is the commitment and interest of people to act together, albeit tacitly, which helps accomplish the social. Thus, while people's participation depends upon their engagement and commitment to being a part of something, to being a member, the ways in which membership is accomplished needs creativity and responsiveness. At the same time, then, that persons who together, through their social knowledge produce and reproduce reality (Berger & Luckmann, 1966), they also perform their membership (Garfinkel, 1967) through their *participation*.

And participation is about much more than simply following rules or conventions which are somehow already settled. Membership is much more complex – we have to locate ourselves in different identities, and perform to multiple audiences. This conundrum is particularly true for nurses. The staff nurse already mentioned, acted, and accounted for her actions, in ways which privileged some kinds of work and patients over others. This idea of privileging suggests that there are always alternatives. For example, at the same time as they want more to be seen as professionals rather than just as 'good women', nurses also need to demonstrate their worth to managers and accountants. Thus nurses cannot rely upon being easily identifiable; rather their visibility is extremely difficult to accomplish.

This problem over the precariousness of identity means that, increasingly, nurses, like other social beings, have to be persuasive. Nurses cannot just act or give an account of themselves; to be compelling, their accounts have to be convincing. In this way, participation is also about making *moves* (Latimer, 1997a, 2000b). In this view, nurses, like Sister cited above, do more than follow rules, they *draw on* discursive grounds, rules and conventions and other materials to give authority to their performances and to legitimate what they do. But not all grounds are equal or available, not all materials will do. Knowing what will give authority, what will do, is all a part of being social.

Conclusion

What I have highlighted is an approach to studying nursing that gets away from the abstractions of theories and models of nursing, although these will enter into nurses' accounts as they offer reasons and justify what they or others do. The approach begins by bringing together two key traditions in qualitative social research. First, an idea that reality is produced and reproduced by participants as they go about their business, and, second, that this going about their business is connected to identity. This is not to suggest that identity is ascribed or given and that action or accounts simply flow from it. Rather, with Goffman (1958), we can understand that identity has always been a precarious business. But I have stretched both the symbolic interactionist and ethnomethodological perspectives to late modern times.

The upshot of these complex ideas about social realities is that identity is becoming increasingly haphazard and problematic (Bauman, 1997). At the same time, the call for individuals to perform their distinctiveness is being intensified (Latimer, 2001). On the one hand, then, there is an intensification for individuals to *perform* their identity, but on the other, the typifications and categories which people participate in to perform their identity are less and less settled. Part of the work of belonging is precisely to show, like Sister and Staff Nurse cited above, that you know how to settle (or unsettle) matters of identity.

My focus, the assessment and care of older patients in an acute adult care unit, helps make this explicit. Here, there is no singular reality, no grand narrative (Lyotard, 1984) to help settle matters, but multiple possibilities for interpretation and conduct. This means that, as researchers, we are not just looking to see how matters are already settled: that is, we are not looking for 'the whole' that, through playing the right part, participants can simply become a part of. Rather, as Purkis, Rudge and Traynor (this volume) have already, in their different ways, suggested, we need to examine how matters are being settled (or unsettled) by people as they go about their business. This applies not only to matters between different groups with different interests, but also within groups and even to individuals themselves. This is because, for groups as well as for individuals, there are competing possibilities for interpretation and conduct, competing narratives, competing agendas.

Thus, in our approaches to researching nursing, at the same time as we need to explore what people as they work and interact make categories mean, we also need to be able to explore how people make meanings 'stick' (Rabinow and Sullivan, 1979) and how they 'dispose' (Munro, 1992; Latimer, 1997a; Strathern, 1999) of meanings. In these ways the approach I am offering here stretches both the symbolic interactionist and ethnomethodological traditions to make explicit issues of power.

Notes

1. By knowing here I do not mean something cognitive. Knowing can be tacit or, as Savage (this volume), argues, embodied.
2. Elsewhere (Latimer, 1999, 2001) I have, drawing on Strathern (1991) and Munro (1996b), suggested that a way to understand and explore the relation between materials, identity and power effects is through the concept of extension.
3. As Strathern (1991) argues, in extension we are ourselves a kind of cultural material – extended through technology and other artefacts.
4. I have used Callon and Latour's (1981; Callon, 1986) ideas of enrolment and translation elsewhere (Latimer, 1995; Robinson *et al.*, 1999) to help theorise how nurses through drawing on particular kinds of technology and other cultural materials align with, and thereby reproduce, managerial and other discursive effects.

References

Bauman, Z. (1997) *Life in Fragments*. Oxford: Blackwell.

Becker, Howard S. (1993) How I learned what a crock was. *Journal of Contemporary Ethnography* **22** (1): 28–35.

Becker, H.S., Geer, B., Hughes, E.C. & Strauss, A.L. (1961) *The Boys in White: Student Culture in a Medical School*. Chicago: University of Chicago Press.

Berger, P. and Luckmann, T. (1966) *The Social Construction of Reality. A Treatise in the Sociology if Knowledge*. Harmondsworth: Penguin (reprinted 1991).

Callon, M. (1986) Some elements of a sociology of translation: domestication of the scallops and the fishermen of St Brieuc Bay. In J. Law (ed.) *Power, Action and Belief: A New Sociology of Knowledge?* Sociological Review Monograph 32. London: Routledge & Kegan Paul, pp. 196–233.

Callon, M. and Latour, B. (1981) Unscrewing the big Leviathan: how actors macro-structure reality and how sociologists help them do so. In K.D. Knorr-Cetain & A. Cicourel (eds) *Advances in Social Theory and Methodology: Toward an Integration of Micro and Macro-Sociologies*. London: Routledge.

Douglas, M. and Baron Isherwood (1980) *The World of Goods: Towards an Anthropology of Consumption*. Harmondsworth: Penguin.

Foucault, M. (1976) *The Birth of the Clinic*. London: Tavistock Press.

Giddens, A. (1984) *The Constitution of Society: Outline of Structuration Theory*. Cambridge: Polity Press (reprinted 1989).

Garfinkel, H. (1967) *Studies in Ethnomethodology*. Englewood Cliffs, NJ: Prentice Hall.

Garfinkel, H. and Sacks, H. (1986) On formal structures of practical actions. In H. Garfinkel (ed.) *Ethnomethodological Studies of Work*. London: Routledge & Kegan Paul (first published 1969).

Geertz, C. (1983) *Local Knowledge*. New York: Basic Books.

Geertz, C. (1993) *The Interpretation of Cultures: Selected Essays*. London: Fontana.

Goffman, E. (1958) *The Presentation of Self in Everyday Life*. University of Edinburgh, Social Sciences Research Centre, Monograph No. 2.

Latimer, J. (1995) The nursing process re-examined: diffusion or translation? *Journal of Advanced Nursing* **22**: 213–20.

Latimer, J. (1997a) Giving patients a future: the constituting of classes in an acute medical unit. *Sociology of Health and Illness* **19** (2): 160–85.

Latimer, J. (1997b) Figuring identities: older people, medicine and time. In A. Jamieson, S. Harper & C. Victor (eds) *Critical Approaches to Ageing and Later Life*. Milton Keynes: Open University Press.

Latimer, J. (1999) The dark at the bottom of the stair: participation and performance of older people in hospital. *Medical Anthropology Quarterly* **13** (2): 186–213.

Latimer, J. (2000a) *The Conduct of Care: Understanding Nursing Practice*. Oxford: Blackwell Science.

Latimer, J. (2000b) Socialising disease: medical categories and inclusion of the aged. *Sociological Review* **48** (3): 383–407.

Latimer, J. (2001) All-consuming passions: materials and subjectivity in the age of enhancement. In N. Lee and R. Munro (eds) *The Consumption of Mass*, Sociological Review Monographs. Oxford: Blackwell.

Latour, B. (1986) The powers of association. In J. Law (ed.) *Power, Action and Belief: A New Sociology of Knowledge?*, Sociological Review Monograph 32. London: Routledge & Kegan Paul, pp. 264–80.

Lyotard, J.F. (1984) *The Post-modern Condition: A Report on Knowledge*. Manchester: Manchester University Press.

Munro, R. (1992) Disposal of the body: upending postmodernism, *Organization and Theatre*. Proceedings of 10th Anniversary SCOS conference, Lancaster University.

Munro, R. (1996a) Alignments and identity-work: the study of accounts and accountability. In R. Munro & J. Mouritsen (eds) *Accountability: Power, Ethos and the Technologies of Managing*. London: Thomson International.

Munro, R. (1996b) The consumption view of self: extension, exchange and identity. In S. Edgell, K. Hetherington & A. Warde (eds) *Consumption Matters*, Sociological Review Monograph. Oxford: Blackwell, pp. 248–73.

Rabinow, P. and Sullivan, W.M. (1979) The interpretive turn: emergence of an approach. In P. Rabinow & W.M. Sullivan (eds) *Interpretive Social Science: A Reader*. Berkeley: University of California Press.

Robinson, J., Avis, M., Latimer, J. & Traynor, M. (1999) *Interdisciplinary Perspectives on Health Policy and Practice: Competing Interests or Complementary Interpretations?* Edinburgh: Harcourt Brace/Elsevier Science.

Strathern, M. (1991) *Partial Connections*. Maryland: Rowman & Littlefield.

Strathern, M. (1992) Writing societies, writing persons. *History of Human Sciences* 5 (1): 5–16.

Strathern, M. (1999) *Property, Substance and Effect: Anthropological Essays on Persons and Things*. London: Athlone Press.

Tyler, S.A. (1986) Post-modern ethnography: from document of the occult to occult document. In J. Clifford & G. Marcus (eds) *Writing Culture: The Poetics and Politics of Ethnography*. Berkeley: California University Press.

Epilogue

In a volume that has set out to bring together some of the leading authors in contemporary nursing and health services research, it would be inappropriate to fold all of them together into a concluding summary. But we hope that the book provides a variety of paths into critical approaches to qualitative research on nursing and health care which others can follow.

We know that these approaches are not simplistic or easy. Rather, throughout the book each author has been at pains to explore nurses', patients' and researchers' relations, not as simply prescribed or determined, but as deeply problematic. This is either because, as Parker and Wiltshire elucidate, nurses engage with otherness in ways that are existentially pressing; or because nurses, patients and researchers, as May has elucidated, perform in the context of wider socio-cultural mores and demands which have their own power effects. Each chapter has helped to show that nursing, and researching, do not, and cannot, stand *outside*. Rather, each author has theorised an approach for exploring how nurses' and researchers' relations with and to others are not just mediated *by* social forms, but actually help accomplish the socio-cultural effects which underpin nursing practice. Even patients' narrative accounts, which seem so personal, are, as Ayres and Poirier have elucidated, social.

Our collective aim has been to offer approaches to research that take the socio-political and cultural conditions of nursing seriously. However, at the same time, each author has been mindful that the experience of doing nursing or of being nursed, or of doing or being researched, is not less meaningful for being socially conditioned. On the contrary, we hope to have shown in the book how understanding socialness can help to produce rigorous and relevant insights into patienthood and health care policy and practice.

Index